Advances in Oral and Maxillofacial Surgery

Editors

JOSE M. MARCHENA
JONATHAN W. SHUM
JONATHAN S. JUNDT

ORAL AND MAXILLOFACIAL SURGERY CLINICS OF NORTH AMERICA

www.oralmaxsurgery.theclinics.com

Consulting Editor
RUI P. FERNANDES

November 2019 • Volume 31 • Number 4

ELSEVIER

1600 John F. Kennedy Boulevard • Suite 1800 • Philadelphia, Pennsylvania, 19103-2899

http://www.oralmaxsurgery.theclinics.com

ORAL AND MAXILLOFACIAL SURGERY CLINICS OF NORTH AMERICA Volume 31, Number 4
November 2019 ISSN 1042-3699, ISBN-13: 978-0-323-70898-2

Editor: John Vassallo; j.vassallo@elsevier.com
Developmental Editor: Laura Fisher

Oral and Maxillofacial Surgery Clinics of North America (ISSN 1042-3699) is published quarterly by Elsevier Inc., 360 Park Avenue South, New York, NY 10010-1710. Months of issue are February, May, August, and November. Business and Editorial Offices: 1600 John F. Kennedy Blvd., Suite 1800, Philadelphia, PA 19103-2899. Periodicals postage paid at New York, NY and additional mailing offices. Subscription prices are $401.00 per year for US individuals, $720.00 per year for US institutions, $100.00 per year for US students and residents, $474.00 per year for Canadian individuals, $863.00 per year for Canadian institutions, $520.00 per year for international individuals, $863.00 per year for international institutions and $235.00 per year for Canadian and foreign students/residents. To receive student/resident rate, orders must be accompanied by name or affiliated institution, date of term, and the *signature* of program/residency coordinator on institution letterhead. Orders will be billed at individual rate until proof of status is received. Foreign air speed delivery is included in all *Clinics* subscription prices. All prices are subject to change without notice. **POSTMASTER:** Send address changes to *Oral and Maxillofacial Surgery Clinics of North America,* Elsevier Periodicals **Customer Service, 11830 Westline Industrial Drive, St. Louis, MO 63146. Tel: 1-800-654-2452 (U.S. and Canada); 314-447-8871 (outside U.S. and Canada). Fax: 314-447-8029. E-mail: journals customerservice-usa@elsevier.com (for print support); journalsonlinesupport-usa@elsevier.com (for online support).**

Reprints. For copies of 100 or more, of articles in this publication, please contact the Commercial Reprints Department, Elsevier Inc., 360 Park Avenue South, New York, NY 10010-1710. Tel.: 212-633-3874; Fax: 212-633-3820; Email: reprints@elsevier.com.

Oral and Maxillofacial Surgery Clinics of North America is covered in *MEDLINE/PubMed* (*Index Medicus*), *Science Citation Index Expanded (SciSearch®)*, *Journal Citation Reports/Science Edition*, and *Current Contents®/Clinical Medicine*.

Contributors

CONSULTING EDITOR

RUI P. FERNANDES, MD, DMD, FACS, FRCS(Ed)
Clinical Professor and Chief, Division of Head and Neck Surgery, Departments of Oral and Maxillofacial Surgery, Neurosurgery, and Orthopaedic Surgery and Rehabilitation, University of Florida Health Science Center, University of Florida College of Medicine, Jacksonville, Florida, USA

EDITORS

JOSE M. MARCHENA, DMD, MD, FACS
Associate Professor, Department of Oral and Maxillofacial Surgery, The University of Texas Health Science Center at Houston, Chief of Oral and Maxillofacial Surgery, Ben Taub Hospital, Houston, Texas, USA

JONATHAN W. SHUM, DDS, MD, FACS, FRCD(C)
Associate Professor, Fellowship Director, Maxillofacial Oncology and Microvascular Reconstruction, Department of Oral and Maxillofacial Surgery, The University of Texas Health Science Center at Houston, Houston, Texas, USA

JONATHON S. JUNDT, DDS, MD, FACS
Assistant Professor, Department of Oral and Maxillofacial Surgery, The University of Texas Health Science Center at Houston, Houston, Texas, USA

AUTHORS

DAVID Y. AHN, DMD
Oral and Maxillofacial Surgeon, David Grant USAF Medical Center, Fairfield, California, USA; United States Air Force, Former Fellow Endoscopic Maxillofacial Surgery, Massachusetts General Hospital, Boston, Massachusetts, USA

DAVID ALFI, DDS, MD
Attending Surgeon, Department of Oral and Maxillofacial Surgery, Houston Methodist Hospital, Houston, Texas, USA; Associate Professor of Clinical Oral and Maxillofacial Surgery, Weill Cornell Medical College, New York, New York, USA

JONATHAN ALFI, MA
Project Specialist, Surgical Planning Laboratory, Department of Oral and Maxillofacial Surgery, Houston Methodist Research Institute, Houston, Texas, USA

SHAHID AZIZ, DMD, MD
Professor, Department of Oral and Maxillofacial Surgery, Rutgers School of Dental Medicine, Newark, New Jersey, USA

JAMES BAKER, DDS
Founder, OMS Partners, Houston, Texas, USA

CALEB BLACKBURN, DDS
Department of Oral and Maxillofacial Surgery,
The University of Tennessee Medical Center,
Knoxville, Tennessee, USA

MATTHEW J. BREIT, DMD
Resident, Department of Oral and Maxillofacial
Surgery, The University of Texas Health
Science Center at Houston, Houston, Texas,
USA

**KAMAL F. BUSAIDY, BDS (Lond), FDSRCS
(Eng), FACS**
Professor, Department of Oral and
Maxillofacial Surgery, The University of Texas
Health Science Center at Houston, Houston,
Texas, USA

MARCUS COUEY, DDS, MD
Surgical Fellow, Head and Neck Oncologic and
Microvascular Reconstructive Surgery,
Providence Portland Medical Center, Portland,
Oregon, USA

NAGI DEMIAN, DDS, MD, FACS
Professor, Department of Oral and
Maxillofacial Surgery, The University of Texas
Health Science Center at Houston, Houston,
Texas, USA

YI DENG, MD
Assistant Professor, Department of
Anesthesiology and Critical Care Medicine,
Baylor College of Medicine, Houston, Texas,
USA

**JAGTAR DHANDA, BSc(Hons), BDS, MFDS
RCS(Eng), MBBS, MRCS(Eng),
FRCS(OMFS), PhD**
Senior Consultant, Maxillofacial/Head and
Neck Surgery, Queen Victoria Hospital, East
Grinstead, United Kingdom

ROBERT EMERY III, DDS
Private Practice, Capital Center for Oral
and Maxillofacial Surgery, Washington, DC,
USA

MOHAMED A. HAKIM, DDS
Endoscopic Maxillofacial Surgery
Fellow, Department of Oral and Maxillofacial
Surgery, Massachusetts General
Hospital, Instructor, Harvard School of
Dental Medicine, Boston, Massachusetts,
USA

ISSA HANNA, DDS
Associate Professor, Department of Oral
and Maxillofacial Surgery, The University of
Texas Health Science Center at Houston,
Chief of Oral and Maxillofacial Surgery,
Lyndon B. Johnson Hospital, Houston, Texas,
USA

JACK HUA, DDS, MD
Resident, Department of Oral and Maxillofacial
Surgery, The University of Texas Health
Science Center at Houston, Houston, Texas,
USA

ANDREW T. HUANG, MD
Assistant Professor, Otolaryngology–Head and
Neck Surgery, Baylor College of Medicine,
Houston, Texas, USA

MICHAEL F. HUANG, DDS, MD
Attending Surgeon, Department of Oral and
Maxillofacial Surgery, Houston Methodist
Hospital, Houston, Texas, USA; Assistant
Professor of Oral and Maxillofacial Surgery,
Weill Cornell Medical College, New York,
New York, USA

JONATHON S. JUNDT, DDS, MD, FACS
Assistant Professor, Department of Oral and
Maxillofacial Surgery, The University of Texas
Health Science Center at Houston, Houston,
Texas, USA

AUSTIN LEAVITT, MS, CFP®
Financial Planner, The Financial Advisory
Group, Houston, Texas, USA

LAITH MAHMOOD, DDS, MD
Private Practice, Parkway Oral Surgery
and Dental Implant Center, Houston, Texas,
USA

VICTORIA A. MAÑÓN, DDS
Resident, Department of Oral and Maxillofacial
Surgery, The University of Texas Health
Science Center at Houston, School of
Dentistry, Houston, Texas, USA

JOSE M. MARCHENA, DMD, MD, FACS
Associate Professor, Department of Oral
and Maxillofacial Surgery, The University of
Texas Health Science Center at Houston,
Chief of Oral and Maxillofacial Surgery,
Ben Taub Hospital, Houston, Texas,
USA

SANDEEP MARKAN, MD
Associate Professor, Department of Anesthesiology and Critical Care Medicine, Baylor College of Medicine, Houston, Texas, USA

JOSEPH P. McCAIN, DMD, FACS
Endoscopic Maxillofacial Surgery Fellowship Director, Department of Oral and Maxillofacial Surgery, Massachusetts General Hospital, Faculty Member, Harvard School of Dental Medicine, Boston, Massachusetts, USA

JAMES C. MELVILLE, DDS, FACS
Oral, Head and Neck Oncology and Microvascular Reconstructive Surgery, Associate Professor, Department of Oral and Maxillofacial Surgery, The University of Texas Health Science Center at Houston, School of Dentistry, Houston, Texas, USA

JOVANY CRUZ NAVARRO, MD
Assistant Professor, Departments of Anesthesiology and Neurosurgery, Baylor College of Medicine, Houston, Texas, USA

NEERAJ PANCHAL, DDS, MD, MA
Assistant Professor, University of Pennsylvania School of Dental Medicine, Section Chief, Penn Presbyterian Medical Center, Section Chief, Philadelphia Veterans Affairs Medical Center, Philadelphia, Pennsylvania, USA

ZACHARY S. PEACOCK, DMD, MD, FACS
Assistant Professor, Department of Oral and Maxillofacial Surgery, Massachusetts General Hospital, Harvard School of Dental Medicine, Boston, Massachusetts, USA

CRAIG PEARL, DDS
Assistant Professor, Department of Oral and Maxillofacial Surgery, The University of Texas Health Science Center at Houston, Houston, Texas, USA

ANDREW P. PERRY, DDS
Resident, Department of Oral and Maxillofacial Surgery, The University of Texas Health Science Center at Houston, Houston, Texas, USA

ARMANDO RETANA, DDS, MD
Private Practice, Capital Center for Oral and Maxillofacial Surgery, Washington, DC, USA

JUSTIN SEAMAN, DDS, MD
Assistant Professor, Department of Oral and Maxillofacial Surgery, The University of Texas Health Science Center at Houston, Houston, Texas, USA

JONATHAN W. SHUM, DDS, MD, FACS, FRCD(C)
Associate Professor, Fellowship Director, Maxillofacial Oncology and Microvascular Reconstruction, Department of Oral and Maxillofacial Surgery, The University of Texas Health Science Center at Houston, Houston, Texas, USA

MARIA J. TROULIS, DDS, MSc, FACS
W.C. Guralnick Professor and Chair, Department of Oral and Maxillofacial Surgery, Massachusetts General Hospital, Harvard School of Dental Medicine, Boston, Massachusetts, USA

DAVID Q. WAN, MD
Associate Professor of Radiology, Department of Diagnostic and Interventional Imaging, McGovern Medical School, The University of Texas Health Science Center at Houston, Houston, Texas, USA

JAMES WILSON, DDS, FACS
Professor Emeritus, Department of Oral and Maxillofacial Surgery, The University of Texas Health Science Center at Houston, Houston, Texas, USA

TIMOTHY CHARLES WOERNLEY III, DDS
Assistant Professor, Department of Oral and Maxillofacial Surgery, The University of Texas Health Science Center at Houston, Houston, Texas, USA

SIMON YOUNG, DDS, MD, PhD
Assistant Professor, Department of Oral and Maxillofacial Surgery, The University of Texas Health Science Center at Houston, School of Dentistry, Houston, Texas, USA

Contributors

SANDEEP MARKAN, MD
Associate Professor, Department of Anesthesiology and Critical Care Medicine, Baylor College of Medicine, Houston, Texas, USA

JOSEPH R. McCAIN, DMD, FACS
Endodontic Maxillofacial Surgery Fellowship Director, Department of Oral and Maxillofacial Surgery, Massachusetts General Hospital, Faculty, Massachusetts General Hospital of Dental Medicine, Boston, Massachusetts, USA

JAMES C. MELVILLE, DDS, FACS
Oral, Head and Neck Oncology and Microvascular Reconstructive Surgery, Associate Professor, Department of Oral and Maxillofacial Surgery, The University of Texas Health Science Center at Houston, School of Dentistry, Houston, Texas, USA

JOVANY CRUZ NAVARRO, MD
Assistant Professor, Departments of Anesthesiology and Neurosurgery, Baylor College of Medicine, Houston, Texas, USA

NEERAJ PANCHAL, DDS, MD, MA
Assistant Professor, University of Pennsylvania School of Dental Medicine; Section Chief, Penn Presbyterian Medical Center, Section Chief, Philadelphia Veterans Affairs Medical Center, Philadelphia, Pennsylvania, USA

ZACHARY S. PEACOCK, DMD, MD, FACS
Assistant Professor, Department of Oral and Maxillofacial Surgery, Massachusetts General Hospital, Harvard School of Dental Medicine, Boston, Massachusetts, USA

CRAIG PEARL, DDS
Assistant Professor, Department of Oral and Maxillofacial Surgery, The University of Texas Health Science Center at Houston, Texas, USA

ANDREW P. McCRAY, DDS
Resident, Department of Oral and Maxillofacial Surgery, The University of Texas Health Science Center at Houston, Houston, Texas, USA

ARMANDO RETANA, DDS, MD
Private Practice, Capital Center for Oral and Maxillofacial Surgery, Washington, DC, USA

JUSTIN SEAMAN, DDS, MD
Assistant Professor, Department of Oral and Maxillofacial Surgery, The University of Texas Health Science Center at Houston, Houston, Texas, USA

JONATHAN W. SHUM, DDS, MD, FACS, FRCD(C)
Associate Professor, Fellowship Director, Microvascular Oncology and Reconstruction, Department of Oral and Maxillofacial Surgery, The University of Texas Health Science Center at Houston, Houston, Texas, USA

MARIA J. TROULIS, DDS, MSc, FACS
W.C. Guralnick Professor and Chief, Department of Oral and Maxillofacial Surgery, Massachusetts General Hospital, Harvard School of Dental Medicine, Boston, Massachusetts, USA

DAVID C. WAN, MD
Associate Professor of Radiology, Department of Diagnostic and Interventional Imaging, McGovern Medical School, The University of Texas Health Science Center at Houston, Houston, Texas, USA

JAMES WILSON, DDS, FACS
Assistant Professor, Department of Oral and Maxillofacial Surgery, The University of Texas Health Science Center at Houston, Houston, Texas, USA

TIMOTHY CHARLES WOERNLEY III, DDS
Assistant Professor, Department of Oral and Maxillofacial Surgery, The University of Texas Health Science Center at Houston, Houston, Texas, USA

SIMON YOUNG, DDS, MD, PhD
Assistant Professor, Department of Oral and Maxillofacial Surgery, The University of Texas Health Science Center at Houston, School of Dentistry, Houston, Texas, USA

Contents

maxillofacial endoscopic techniques are used for access to the ramus condyle unit, maxillary sinus, zygoma, orbit, temporomandibular joint, and salivary ductal system. Although endoscopic techniques are also used in facial cosmetic surgery, this discussion focuses on noncosmetic procedures.

Benign cysts and neoplasms of the maxillofacial region can vary in behavior, with some growing rapidly and resulting in destruction of surrounding structures. Despite their benign histology, many require often-morbid treatment to prevent recurrence of these lesions. Several less invasive and adjunctive medical treatments have been developed to lessen the morbidity of surgical treatment. As the molecular and genomic pathogenesis of these lesions is better understood, more directed treatments may lessen the burden for patients.

For several decades, the multidisciplinary field of tissue engineering has striven to improve conventional methods of dental, oral, and craniofacial rehabilitation for millions of people annually. Several bone tissue engineering strategies are now readily available in the clinic. Enrichment of autologous products, growth factors, and combination approaches are discussed as ways to enhance the surgeon's traditional armamentarium. Lastly, cutting-edge research such as customized 3-dimensional printed bone scaffolds, tissue engineering strategies for volumetric muscle loss, and temporomandibular joint disc and condyle engineering are briefly discussed as future applications.

This article summarizes the current use of patient-specific implants in oral and maxillofacial surgery.

Managing an oral and maxillofacial surgery (OMS) practice has undergone dramatic changes. Electronic health records, privacy laws, revenue cycle management, online marketing, and the rise of dental service organizations (DSOs) present increased daily complexity for oral and maxillofacial surgeons in private practice, hospital-based employees, and academic surgeons. This article is structured to discuss the role of DSOs, private equity in OMS, online practice marketing, accounting and tax considerations, and modern essentials of practice management.

During surgery, one of the primary functions of the anesthesiologist is to monitor the patient and ensure safe and effective conduct of anesthesia to provide the optimum operating conditions. Standard guidelines for perioperative monitoring have been firmly established by the American Society of Anesthesiologists. However, in recent years, new advances in technology has led to the development of many new monitoring modalities, especially involving the neurologic and cardiovascular systems. This article presents a targeted review to discuss the functions and limitations of these new monitors and how they are applied in the modern operating room setting.

ORAL AND MAXILLOFACIAL SURGERY CLINICS OF NORTH AMERICA

SERIES OF RELATED INTEREST

Atlas of the Oral and Maxillofacial Surgery Clinics
www.oralmaxsurgeryatlas.theclinics.com

Dental Clinics
www.dental.theclinics.com

THE CLINICS ARE NOW AVAILABLE ONLINE!
Access your subscription at:
www.theclinics.com

Preface
The Evolution of Technological Advancements in Oral and Maxillofacial Surgery

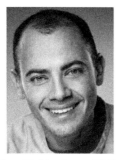

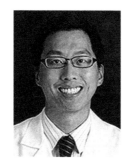

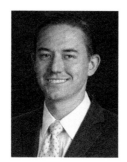

Jose M. Marchena, DMD, MD, FACS

Jonathan W. Shum, DDS, MD, FACS, FRCD(C)

Jonathon S. Jundt, DDS, MD, FACS

Editors

It has been suggested that we are what we repeatedly do, and excellence, then, is not an act but a habit.[1] This is irreconcilable with Heraclitus of Ephesus' notion that change is the only constant.[2] Surgeons must possess a duality of nature that in 1 instance embraces habit to effect consistent results in the surgical theater and in the other allows for ingenuity to solve immediate challenges. A purely stepwise approach to surgery would yield devastating results when biology fails to follow the rules. This series provides information about technological advances that may become routine practice in the coming years.

Everett Rogers observed that technological advances are born in the midst of innovators, refined by early adopters, popularized by an early majority, standardized by the late majority, and occasionally phased out by laggards.[3] Proximity to hubs of ingenuity, whether intentional or by chance, provides opportunities for clinicians to innovate or become early adopters in a technology. Social and economic factors may incline clinicians toward late majority adoption of new concepts. Personality, predictability, and risk tolerance further influence a practitioner's willingness to alter their current practice.

The editors' intent for this series is to review and summarize selected technological advancements in Oral and Maxillofacial Surgery that are either gaining popularity or infrequently discussed in our specialty. Given the rapidly changing trends in practice management, evolving management strategies and technologies used in practice management are also reviewed. We would like to thank the authors for their contributions and for unselfishly sharing their knowledge and expertise. It is our hope that this information presented within a single source will prove useful to all practicing oral and maxillofacial surgeons, including those in training.

Jose M. Marchena, DMD, MD, FACS
Department of Oral and Maxillofacial Surgery
The University of Texas
Health Science Center at Houston
6560 Fannin Street
Suite 1900, Floor 19th
Houston, TX 77030, USA

Jonathan W. Shum, DDS, MD, FACS, FRCD(C)
Maxillofacial Oncology and
Microvascular Reconstruction
Department of Oral and Maxillofacial Surgery
The University of Texas
Health Science Center at Houston
6560 Fannin Street
Suite 1900, Floor 19th
Houston, TX 77030, USA

Oral Maxillofacial Surg Clin N Am 31 (2019) xi–xii
https://doi.org/10.1016/j.coms.2019.08.002
1042-3699/19/© 2019 Published by Elsevier Inc.

Jonathon S. Jundt, DDS, MD, FACS
Department of Oral and Maxillofacial Surgery
The University of Texas
Health Science Center at Houston
6560 Fannin Street
Suite 1900, Floor 19th
Houston, TX 77030, USA

E-mail addresses:
jose.m.marchena@uth.tmc.edu (J.M. Marchena)
jonathan.shum@uth.tmc.edu (J.W. Shum)
jonathon.jundt@uth.tmc.edu (J.S. Jundt)

REFERENCES

1. Durant W. The story of philosophy: the lives and opinions of the great philosophers of the western world. New York: Simon and Schuster; 1961.
2. Mark JJ. Heraclitus of Ephesus. Ancient History Encyclopedia. Available at: https://www.ancient.eu/Heraclitus_of_Ephesos/. Accessed March 21, 2019.
3. Rogers EM. Diffusion of innovations. 5th edition. New York: Free Press; 2003.

Virtual Surgical Planning in Oral and Maxillofacial Surgery

Jack Hua, DDS, MD[a], Shahid Aziz, DMD, MD[b], Jonathan W. Shum, DDS, MD[a],*

KEYWORDS

- Virtual surgical planning • Maxillofacial reconstruction • Maxillofacial trauma • Jaw reconstruction
- Computer-aided design • Computer aided manufacture • Imaging modality • Data acquisition

KEY POINTS

- Virtual surgical planning is a process that begins at the collection of imaging data.
- A treatment plan is derived through the manipulation imaging data to visualize and predict an effective surgical approach and/or reconstructive plan.
- Advantages for the use of virtual surgical planning include improved surgical efficiency, and reconstructions to have a higher degree of accuracy when compared between preoperative and postoperative imaging.

INTRODUCTION

Since the 1980s, systematic application of computer aided design and manufacturing in health care has revolutionized diagnostic and interventional medicine.[1] The digital manipulation of large-scale imaging data in 3 dimensions, specifically virtual surgical planning (VSP), provides the ability to reproduce detailed anatomic models, and to fabricate surgical guides and custom implants.[2] These advancements have become an invaluable tool for oral and maxillofacial surgeons. The success of these virtually planned cases depends on each step of the workflow process: choice of image modality, data acquisition, patient workup, virtual planning session, and surgical execution. Although each step of the case is critical, meticulous effort placed in the early planning phases will increase the likelihood of success in the operating room.

IMAGING MODALITY

Selecting the appropriate imaging modality is an important initial step and depends on the advantages in spatial and contrast resolution. Spatial resolution is the ability for an image modality to differentiate between 2 separate objects in a radiographic image (ie, a nerve canal within the mandible) (**Fig. 1**), whereas contrast resolution is the ability to differentiate image intensities between 2 areas (ie, fat stranding vs normal adipose tissue).[3] Computed tomography (CT) scanning has high spatial resolution, but is somewhat limited in contrast resolution. For this reason, CT scans are ideal for oral and maxillofacial cases because they often involve hard tissue interventions, such as surgery on the bones and teeth. Similarly, cone beam CT has many advantages when used in the appropriate surgical setting. Cone beam CT scans offer high spatial resolution with less radiation exposure compared with CT scans, but at

Disclosure Statement: The authors have nothing to disclose.
[a] Department of Oral and Maxillofacial Surgery, The University of Texas Health Science Center at Houston, 6560 Fannin Street, Suite 1900, Houston, TX 77030, USA; [b] Department of Oral and Maxillofacial Surgery, Rutgers School of Dental Medicine, 90 Bergen Street, Suite 7700, Newark, NJ 07103, USA
* Corresponding author.
E-mail address: jonathan.shum@uth.tmc.edu

Oral Maxillofacial Surg Clin N Am 31 (2019) 519–530
https://doi.org/10.1016/j.coms.2019.07.011

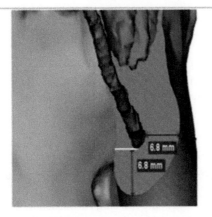
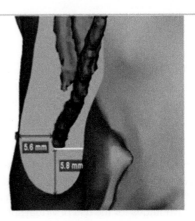

Fig. 1. CT-rendered inferior alveolar nerve measurements. (*Courtesy of* 3D Systems, Rock Hill, SC.)

the cost of poor contrast resolution.[4] For a detailed evaluation of soft tissue structures, MRIs have far superior contrast resolution when compared with CT scans.[5] As an additional method to improve the resolution of surface structures, 3-dimensional (3D) laser scanning is now used to provide the fine detail necessary to facilitate procedures where meticulous detail, such as the ridges and grooves of teeth, are necessary. For example, the fabrication of occlusal splints used in orthognathic surgery can be created from data acquired from laser topography; in turn, traditional stone models are no longer necessary (**Figs. 2** and **3**). These images are acquired with a 3D laser topography scanner and stored as a stereolithography file. The stereolithography data will undergo Digital

Imaging and Communications in Medicine (DICOM) encapsulation to create a reliable superimposed 3D image to be used in conjunction with DICOM data to create an accurate virtual representation of an object, that is, dentition and gingiva. Kau and colleagues[6] examined facial scans of 40 patients and found that 90% of the cases had less than 1.0 mm of error. Schendel and colleagues[7] also evaluated the accuracy of 3D facial scanning in orthognathic surgery and measured 18 cephalometric landmarks among 28 patients and found all of the superimposed landmarks were no more than a 0.55 mm apart. The aforementioned merged DICOM/stereolithography images can be used to accurately facilitate virtual maxillofacial skeletal osteotomies and movements based on both soft and hard tissue reference points (see **Fig. 3**; **Fig. 4**).

DATA ACQUISITION

The foundation of successful surgical planning depends on the ability of the acquired dataset to replicate anatomic detail and translate into virtual modeling and editing software to permit surgical planning. For this reason, the radiographic data are stored in DICOM format so they can be universally shared and used in health care for a variety of applications. With respect to VSP, DICOM data can undergo processing that will allow translation into 3D objects, which can then be manipulated in additional software for VSP. Software programs such as *Materialize Mimics* can readily convert DICOM images to a 3D object file type that will

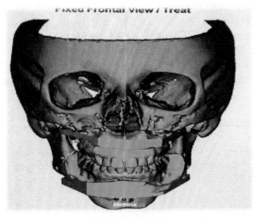

Fig. 2. Superimposition of stone casts on CT scan.

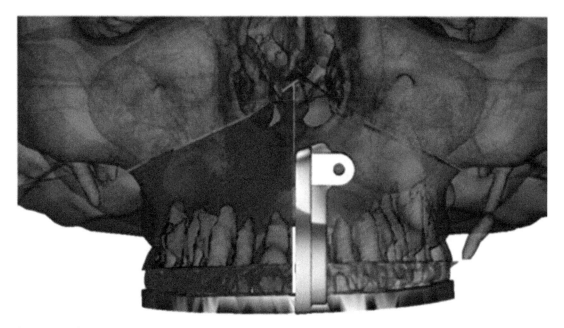

Fig. 3. Virtual cutting guide based on osteotomies.

then allow for surgical planning or fabrication of the model via a 3D printer (**Fig. 5**). Computer-assisted design software such as *Proplan* by Materialise (Leuven, Belgium) or *Sculpt* and *Geomagic Freeform* by 3D Systems (Rock Hill, SC) are commercially available for use. Alternatively, one could collaborate directly with a vendor to facilitate the data rendering, planning, and manufacturing stages of VSP. Access to an engineer is widely available, and video conferencing

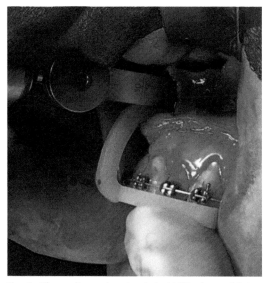

Fig. 4. Three-dimensional–printed VSP-planned interdental osteotomy cutting guide.

for treatment plans has become as convenient as using one's mobile phone to complete the virtual planning (**Fig. 6**). These applications have the ability to edit, render, and analyze the 3D objects to a precision of 0.1 mm and to produce a file that can then be forwarded to additional programs to fabricate the guides or to create hardware.[8] Common with these programs is the use of haptic devices to provide the user with the sense of touch to assist in the interaction with the virtual objects. Most hard tissue reconstruction cases require high-resolution CT scans, with specifications for the image slices ranging from 0.625 to 1.500 mm thin.[9] Although thinner slices do capture more detail into the dataset, Hashemi and colleagues[10] examined temporal bone length obtained from a 1 mm-sliced CT versus during surgery and found that the radiographic measurements were reliably similar to intraoperative ones. In contrast, Rajati and colleagues[10,11] found that 1 mm-sliced CT imaging also provide reliable detail in locating facial nerve injury in temporal bone trauma. To limit radiation exposure and optimize effectiveness, 1 mm-slice CT scans are often adequate for oral and maxillofacial bony reconstruction. An alternative to CT imaging is the use of high-resolution MRIs. The strength of the magnets are measured in Tesla (T), which are proportionate to the ability to create high-resolution images.[12] Most hospitals use 1.5 T and 3 T MRI systems that produce up to 5 and 3 mm slices, respectively. High-powered 7 T MRI systems can produce submillimeter slices; however, these are currently not widely available in

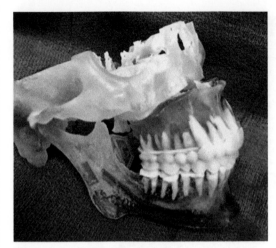

Fig. 5. Stereolithic printed model.

the United States owing to costs.[12] More recently, black bone MRI techniques have been developed to be a nonionizing alternative to CT scans for creating 3D printed guides in the pediatric patient population.[13] Suchyta and colleagues[14] compared osteotomies in cadavers from preoperative guides fabricated from black bone MRI scans versus CT scans and found no statistical difference in accuracy between the 2 imaging modalities. Hoving and colleagues[15] presented 2 successful cases of mandibular resection from an MRI-based 3D-surgical plan, thus, demonstrating that MRI-based VSP is a feasible alternative with foreseeable benefits in the pediatric population.[14] These methods to obtain data apply to all applications of maxillofacial surgery, including the management of pathology, trauma, and dentofacial abnormalities. Ultimately, whether planning for a tumor resection, panfacial reconstruction, or orthognathic surgery, the acquired anatomic detail

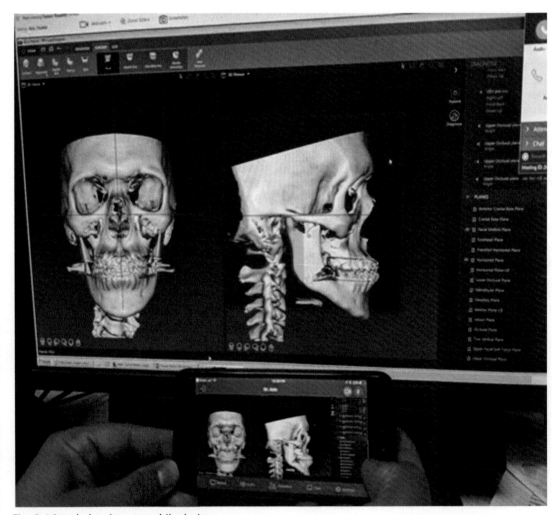

Fig. 6. Virtual planning on mobile device.

must be digitized and translated into virtual planning software to create surgical guides and custom implants to facilitate a successful surgical outcome. Every inaccuracy accumulated at each step can negatively affect the overall surgical case.

APPLICATION
Maxillofacial Trauma

VSP provides the surgeon an opportunity to minimize the uncertainty associated with surgery. The ability to visualize resection margins and to design reconstructive strategies is a significant benefit to management of facial trauma, craniofacial surgery, and pathology. In the setting of maxillofacial trauma, VSP allows for the fabrication of custom implants.[16] Midface trauma, including the orbit, has benefit most from the advancements in VSP and navigation. A systematic review by Azarmehr and colleagues[17] clearly defines the advantages of computer-guided techniques over conventional nonguided methods for the management of facial trauma. VSP coupled with surgical navigation is noted to be most useful in orbital reconstruction owing to the limitations in surgical access, the relationship to surrounding vital structures, and the strict demand for function and aesthetics of the eye.[18] Cai and colleagues[19] conducted a prospective study that compared ophthalmologic complications (ie, diplopia, infraorbital hypoesthesia, ophthalmoplegia, and enophthalmos) of 58 patients undergoing orbital reconstruction and found that the VSP-guided group had significantly fewer complications than the conventional (control) group. Similarly, Bly and colleagues[20] analyzed 90 patients undergoing consecutive complex orbital repairs and found that VSP-guided orbital reconstruction had statistically significant improvement in diplopia severity and a decrease in the incidence of revision surgery when compared with nonguided techniques. In essence, the advantages of VSP in midface reconstruction, especially orbital repair help improve outcomes of complex maxillofacial trauma.

Orthognathic Surgery

VSP is ideal for orthognathic surgical planning as well—it provides for precise and predictable movements of the maxillofacial skeleton in an efficient and effective manner compared with conventional model surgery.[21] No longer is it necessary for patients, technicians, and surgeons to undergo numerous dental impressions, face bow measurements, and laboratory workups. Numerous opportunities for error and inaccuracies exist in the traditional orthognathic workup. Many if not all of the problems associated with the

onerous sequence of a traditional orthognathic workup can be avoided in a VSP-guided workflow.[21] Azarmehr and colleagues[17] summarized orthognathic VSP literature to suggest unanimous support for VSP and navigation guidance in orthognathic surgery owing to its accuracy and efficiency in preoperative planning compared with conventional model surgery. Additionally, numerous studies evaluating the effectiveness of a VSP-driven workup conclude this method to be as effective and accurate when comparing pretreatment and post-treatment cephalometric measurements, with the added benefit of being more efficient with the use of time and resources.[22,23] Resnick and colleagues[24] further examined operative time and cost of bimaxillary surgeries of 43 patients to show that operative time and costs were significantly higher in all the patients with conventional orthognathic workup compared with VSP. These findings are significant because a prolonged operative time is closely correlated with increased postoperative complications.[25,26] The advantages of VSP are clear and established; a standard orthognathic VSP workflow is outlined in **Fig. 7**.

Pathology and Reconstruction

VSP is used extensively in the management of maxillofacial pathology for its ability to virtually visualize pathology and to provide guidance on the location of resection margins.[26–28] The application of guided osteotomies is most beneficial in surgical resections of the midface and for large tumors that have deformed anatomic landmarks (**Figs. 8** and **9**). Characteristics of midface pathology include the difficulties in removing tumors within the maxillary sinus or nasal cavity, where osteotomies are often performed without direct visualization of the tumor. Surgical planning allows for such resections to be performed with greater confidence when visual cues are absent. Furthermore, the proximity to vital structures of the skull base can be accounted for and designed into the cutting guides to prevent inadvertent injury. The coupling of real-time 3D navigation and VSP further enhances these advantages to provide immediate feedback to confirm position of guides and planned osteotomies (**Figs. 10** and **11**). Recent studies demonstrate the benefits of VSP and navigation by reporting a statistically significant difference in 91% of patients in obtaining a clear margin along deep tumor margins with an accuracy of less than 5 mm difference of the actual resection margin compared with the planned margin.[29,30] Bernstein and colleagues[31] and Foley and colleagues[32] compared 224 osteotomies

---

Data Collection

1. Obtain intraoral and extraoral photographs with a standardized background (white or blue wall)
2. Fabricate stone or digital models (intraoral scans) in reproducible centric occlusion
3. Deliver data to processing center for rendering (digital upload or physical media)
4. Often stone casts are sent with digital scans as a reference mark to the final occlusion
5. Though optional, casts are particular helpful in segmental surgical planning

Pre-Planning

1. Stone models are superimposed with CT images to check for inaccuracies
2. Once verified, scans are imported into digital cephalometric program such as Dolphin
3. Cephalometric points and planned osteotomies are imported into the digitized facial skeleton
4. Coordinate planning session with surgeon, engineer, and possibly orthodontist

Planning Session (Digital Model Surgery)

1. First, assess for maxillary cant and maxillary dental and facial midline (refer to clinical photos)
2. Le Fort osteotomy is virtually placed based on anatomical landmarks (i.e. canine apices)
3. If required, interdental maxillary osteotomies can be placed at this time
4. Cephalometric measurements are placed in the lateral view (SNA, SNB, maxillary depth, etc.)
5. Determine vertical position of maxilla based on clinical photos
6. Once the maxilla is in ideal position, the mandible can be placed into class 1 canine occlusion
7. The type of mandible osteotomy (SSO vs. VRO) should be made known to all planning members
8. A genioplasty can be virtually executed at this point, if necessary

Manufacturing Considerations

1. Osteotomy guides are typically based on occlusal surfaces for stability
2. Occlusal splints are fabricated to guide the final position of the osteotomy segments
3. Stereolithic models allow evaluation of critical landmarks (i.e. neurovascular bundle)

Fig. 7. Orthognathic surgery workflow. SNA, Sella Nasion, A; SNB, Sella Nasion, B; SSO, Sagittal Split Osteotomy; VRO, Vertical Ramus Osteotomy.

made with 3D-navigated virtual cutting guides and 224 without navigation and found that osteotomies made with 3D navigation to be more accurate in distance, pitch, and roll. Although more studies are needed to compare 3D navigation and VSP-based resection techniques, the potential is evident in its application in the management of pathology.

Parallel to the extirpation of tumors is the reconstruction of said defect. VSP has made a significant impact on all aspects of reconstruction. It has made reconstruction a streamline process

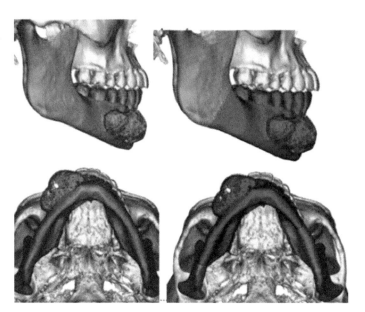

Fig. 8. The resection margins are defined and viewed on a virtual model.

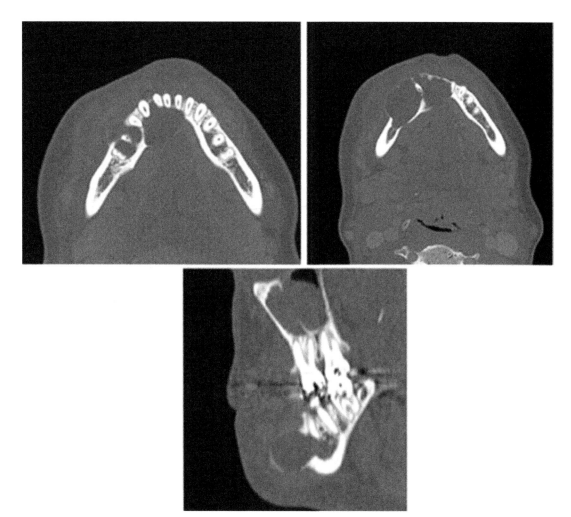

Fig. 9. The corresponding defined resection margins can referenced onto the original CT imaging to ensure clearance from the identified tumor.

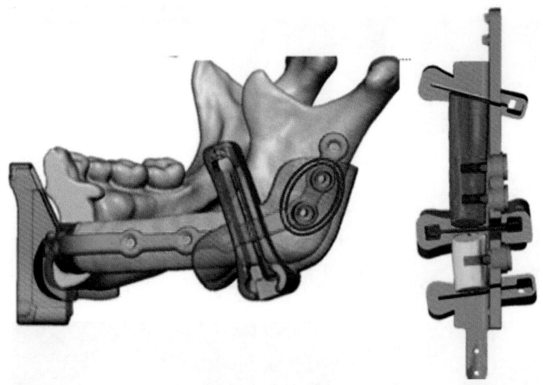

Fig. 10. Virtual planned cutting guides with predictive holes to facilitate hardware placement (*blue circle*). Right fibula bone segments secured to cutting template, with virtual fibula and estimated endosseous implants to be placed while in situ of donor site.

that is cost effective, without jeopardizing outcomes or increasing complication rates.[33] VSP-guided surgery is reportedly 60 to 120 minutes faster in microvascular tissue transfers using a bony donor site, such as the fibula osteocutaneous free flap, when compared with nonguided surgery.[34,35] Complex bony constructs to restore the midface and defects of the anterior mandible

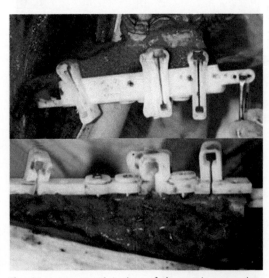

Fig. 11. Intraoperative view of the cutting template secured to the fibula osteocutaneous free flap while in situ in leg. Right – endosseous implants are placed with cutting template.

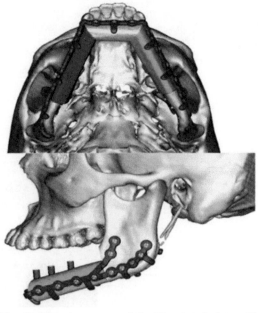

Fig. 12. Virtual construct of the 3D-printed plate with registration tabs and planned dental implants.

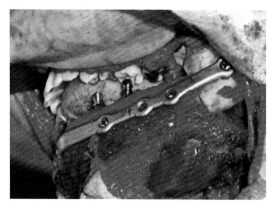

Fig. 13. The fibula osteocutaneous flap forms a neo-mandible as it is secured to the native remaining mandible by reconstruction plate. The endosseous implants are precisely positioned based on VSP.

demonstrate the highest degree of accuracy and precision with the use of VSP.[33,36,37] Additionally, fewer nonunions are reported and bone-to-bone contact is optimized between osteotomy segments. Delayed and immediate dental rehabilitation with endosseous implants have also become possible because of the precision of VSP-guided reconstructions. This has permitted more reconstructions of the jaws to attain a functional dental rehabilitation either immediately or in a staged manner (**Figs. 12** and **13**). Approximately 40% to 50% of patients who have undergone microvascular reconstruction of a jaw defect and dental implant placement obtain a functional dental prosthesis compared with only 15% to 20% in patients who have undergone non–VSP-guided reconstructions of the jaws.[38–40] Before VSP, the inability to accurately predict the location of

---

Data Collection

1. High resolution CT @1mm slices or less
2. Obtain DICOM files (usually <48hrs of scan) and load onto physical media (CD, data drive, etc.)
3. Upload data to processing center for rendering (often manufacturing company)
4. Data reviewed by engineers and prepared for virtual planning session (usually within 24–48hrs)
5. Coordinate planning session with surgeon, engineer, and manufacturing representative

↓

VSP: Tumor resection

1. Examine lesion(s) in virtual three-dimensional space
2. Review tumor on imaging: Assess extent of tumor, proximity to vital structures
3. Define desired margins for resection

↓

Cutting Template Design

1. Consider access to the mandible/maxilla. Consider relevant anatomical landmarks and reference points
2. Consideration of metal vs. plastic guides.
3. Addition of notches, tabs, or markers to facilitate accurate placement of guides
4. Predictive fixation holes to guide the plan for reconstruction hardware

Fig. 14. Oral and maxillofacial jaw resection workflow.

the fibula segments and their relationship to the opposing arch severely limited the placement or function of dental implants.

These advantages derived from VSP will continue to evolve and refine the efficiency and precision of complex surgeries of the head and neck. An example workflow of the extirpation of a tumor (squamous cell carcinoma) (**Fig. 14**) and (fibula free flap) reconstruction (**Fig. 15**) is provided.

LIMITATIONS

Although VSP can improve the outcomes of many complex and technically challenging surgeries, it has limitations that are currently beyond the surgeons' control. Barriers to the effective use of VSP are associated with the inherent delays associated with current manufacturing capabilities and human error. On average, the authors' experience with the turnover between VSP planning session to delivery of implant/guides can range between 7 to 14 days for pre-bent and milled hardware, whereas 3D printed plates and laser sintered hardware can be produced in 14 to 17 days. These limitations are due to the logistics involved in the processing, quality control, and transportation of the prostheses. Several options are available to

---

Reconstructive Planning

1. Review defect projection, based on tumor resection plan
2. Determine composition of tissue for reconstruction: composite vs. bone only:
   a. Vascularized vs. Non-vascularized Graft
3. Determine donor site
   1. Vascularized graft: review vascular studies
4. Determine construct for reconstruction of defect
   1. Consider shape of defect, multi segment reconstruction
   2. Positioning for ideal endosseous dental implant placement
5. Consider relevant anatomical landmarks to assist in proper placement of guide

Hardware Design

1. Custom reconstruction hardware requires CT scans with <3 mm slices (preferred)
2. Custom hardware offers increased density and strength than compared to malleable plates of similar thickness
3. Determine type of plate, plate design, and thickness
4. Determine number of screws for fixation
5. Consider incorporation of registration tabs to assist in seating of hardware.
6. Determine date for delivery of guides and hardware

Manufacturing Considerations

1. Milled plates offer greatest strength; however, have limited design shapes (cut out of 1 block)
2. Selective Laser Sintering (SLS) plates can obtain any shape with added tabs, cribs, mesh, etc.

Fig. 15. Oral and maxillofacial reconstruction workflow.

reduce the turnaround time, through the use of in office 3D printers and institutional resources.

Human error is inevitable and can be applied to every aspect of the VSP process. Potential sources of inaccuracies in the preoperative setting would be related to miscommunication between physicians, technicians, and assistants. The coordination of care is essential for effective health care delivery; however, the specifications for imaging often are not conveyed accurately to the radiology center or the data may not be processed adequately, and the resulting effect is DICOM files that are not compatible with the planning software. Subsequently, the discovery of inadequate data leads to delays relating to the need for additional imaging and use of resources. In the operating room, surgeon error can be related to the application of guides to designated reference points. Errors may occur if one is not familiar with the hardware and instruments or if a surgeon overlooks details of the surgical plan. The most common point for error is the application of the resection guide or of the reconstruction guide to the donor site, followed by inadequate technique, such as performing an osteotomy at the wrong angle. These nuances can result in deviations from the ideal outcome; however, they serve more as sources of frustration than significant adverse events.

Virtual surgical planning will continue to improve, and methods to acquire and process patient data will become more refined. Meticulous attention to each step is necessary to ensure a positive outcome. Future trends will likely include wide spread availability of 3D printing and manufacturing technology and an increasing number of surgeons taking on the role of the engineer.

REFERENCES

1. Doi K. Computer-aided diagnosis in medical imaging: historical review, current status and future potential. Comput Med Imaging Graph 2007;31(4–5): 198–211.
2. Efanov JI, Roy AA, Huang KN, et al. Virtual surgical planning: the pearls and pitfalls. Plast Reconstr Surg Glob Open 2018;6(1):e1443.
3. Allisy-Roberts P, Williams J. Farr's physics for medical imaging. New York: W.B. Saunders Company; 2007.
4. Pauwels R, Beinsberger J, Stamatakis H, et al. Comparison of spatial and contrast resolution for conebeam computed tomography scanners. Oral Surg Oral Med Oral Pathol Oral Radiol 2012;114(1): 127–35.
5. Lin E, Alessio A. What are the basic concepts of temporal, contrast, and spatial resolution in cardiac CT? J Cardiovasc Comput Tomogr 2009;3(6):403–8.
6. Kau CH, Richmond S, Zhurov AI, et al. Reliability of measuring facial morphology with a 3-dimensional laser scanning system. Am J Orthod Dentofacial Orthop 2005;128(4):424–30.
7. Schendel SA, Jacobson R, Khalessi S. 3-dimensional facial simulation in orthognathic surgery: is it accurate? J Oral Maxillofac Surg 2013;71(8): 1406–14.
8. ProPlan CMF 3.0.1 instructions for software use. Plymouth (MI): Materialise Inc; 2017. p. 3.
9. Cernigliaro JG. ACR practice parameter for performing and Interpreting diagnostic computed tomography (CT). Reston (VA): Radiology ACo; 2014. p. 2.
10. Hashemi J, Rajati M, Rezayani L, et al. Temporal bone measurements; a comparison between rendered spiral CT and surgery. Iran J Radiol 2014;11(3):e9400.
11. Rajati M, Pezeshki Rad M, Irani S, et al. Accuracy of high-resolution computed tomography in locating facial nerve injury sites in temporal bone trauma. Eur Arch Otorhinolaryngol 2014;271(8):2185–9.
12. Petridou N, Italiaander M, van de Bank BL, et al. Pushing the limits of high-resolution functional MRI using a simple high-density multi-element coil design. NMR Biomed 2013;26(1):65–73.
13. Eley KA, Watt-Smith SR, Golding SJ. "Black Bone" MRI: a novel imaging technique for 3D printing. Dentomaxillofac Radiol 2017;46(3):20160407.
14. Suchyta MA, Gibreel W, Hunt CH, et al. Using black bone magnetic resonance imaging in craniofacial virtual surgical planning: a comparative cadaver study. Plast Reconstr Surg 2018;141(6): 1459–70.
15. Hoving AM, Kraeima J, Schepers RH, et al. Optimisation of three-dimensional lower jaw resection margin planning using a novel Black Bone magnetic resonance imaging protocol. PLoS One 2018;13(4): e0196059.
16. Herford AS, Miller M, Lauritano F, et al. The use of virtual surgical planning and navigation in the treatment of orbital trauma. Chin J Traumatol 2017; 20(1):9–13.
17. Azarmehr I, Stokbro K, Bell RB, et al. Surgical navigation: a systematic review of indications, treatments, and outcomes in oral and maxillofacial surgery. J Oral Maxillofac Surg 2017;75(9): 1987–2005.
18. Jansen J, Schreurs R, Dubois L, et al. The advantages of advanced computer-assisted diagnostics and three-dimensional preoperative planning on implant position in orbital reconstruction. J Craniomaxillofac Surg 2018;46(4):715–21.
19. Cai EZ, Koh YP, Hing EC, et al. Computer-assisted navigational surgery improves outcomes in orbital reconstructive surgery. J Craniofac Surg 2012; 23(5):1567–73.

20. Bly RA, Chang SH, Cudejkova M, et al. Computer-guided orbital reconstruction to improve outcomes. JAMA Facial Plast Surg 2013;15(2):113–20.

21. Zhang N, Liu S, Hu Z, et al. Accuracy of virtual surgical planning in two-jaw orthognathic surgery: comparison of planned and actual results. Oral Surg Oral Med Oral Pathol Oral Radiol 2016;122(2):143–51.

22. Van den Bempt M, Liebregts J, Maal T, et al. Toward a higher accuracy in orthognathic surgery by using intraoperative computer navigation, 3D surgical guides, and/or customized osteosynthesis plates: a systematic review. J Craniomaxillofac Surg 2018;46(12):2108–19.

23. Zinser MJ, Sailer HF, Ritter L, et al. A paradigm shift in orthognathic surgery? A comparison of navigation, computer-aided designed/computer-aided manufactured splints, and "classic" intermaxillary splints to surgical transfer of virtual orthognathic planning. J Oral Maxillofac Surg 2013;71(12):2151.e1-21.

24. Resnick CM, Inverso G, Wrzosek M, et al. Is there a difference in cost between standard and virtual surgical planning for orthognathic surgery? J Oral Maxillofac Surg 2016;74(9):1827–33.

25. Cheng H, Chen BP, Soleas IM, et al. Prolonged operative duration increases risk of surgical site infections: a systematic review. Surg Infect (Larchmt) 2017;18(6):722–35.

26. Chim H, Wetjen N, Mardini S. Virtual surgical planning in craniofacial surgery. Semin Plast Surg 2014;28(3):150–8.

27. Shen Y, Sun J, Li J, et al. Special considerations in virtual surgical planning for secondary accurate maxillary reconstruction with vascularised fibula osteomyocutaneous flap. J Plast Reconstr Aesthet Surg 2012;65(7):893–902.

28. Kim NK, Kim HY, Kim HJ, et al. Considerations and protocols in virtual surgical planning of reconstructive surgery for more accurate and esthetic neo-mandible with deep circumflex iliac artery free flap. Maxillofac Plast Reconstr Surg 2014;36(4):161–7.

29. Tarsitano A, Ricotta F, Baldino G, et al. Navigation-guided resection of maxillary tumours: the accuracy of computer-assisted surgery in terms of control of resection margins - a feasibility study. J Craniomaxillofac Surg 2017;45(12):2109–14.

30. Ricotta F, Cercenelli L, Battaglia S, et al. Navigation-guided resection of maxillary tumors: can a new volumetric virtual planning method improve outcomes in terms of control of resection margins? J Craniomaxillofac Surg 2018;46(12):2240–7.

31. Bernstein JM, Daly MJ, Chan H, et al. Accuracy and reproducibility of virtual cutting guides and 3D-navigation for osteotomies of the mandible and maxilla. PLoS ONE 2017;12(3). e0173111.

32. Foley BD, Thayer WP, Honeybrook A, et al. Mandibular reconstruction using computer-aided design and computer-aided manufacturing: an analysis of surgical results. J Oral Maxillofac Surg 2013;71(2):e111–9.

33. Toto JM, Chang EI, Agag R, et al. Improved operative efficiency of free fibula flap mandible reconstruction with patient-specific, computer-guided preoperative planning. Head Neck 2015;37(11):1660–4.

34. Zweifel DF, Simon C, Hoarau R, et al. Are virtual planning and guided surgery for head and neck reconstruction economically viable? J Oral Maxillofac Surg 2015;73(1):170–5.

35. Chang EI, Jenkins MP, Patel SA, et al. Long-term operative outcomes of preoperative computed tomography-guided virtual surgical planning for osteocutaneous free flap mandible reconstruction. Plast Reconstr Surg 2016;137(2):619–23.

36. Antony AK, Chen WF, Kolokythas A, et al. Use of virtual surgery and stereolithography-guided osteotomy for mandibular reconstruction with the free fibula. Plast Reconstr Surg 2011;128(5):1080–4.

37. Liu XJ, Gui L, Mao C, et al. Applying computer techniques in maxillofacial reconstruction using a fibula flap: a messenger and an evaluation method. J Craniofac Surg 2009;20(2):372–7.

38. Avraham T, Franco P, Brecht LE, et al. Functional outcomes of virtually planned free fibula flap reconstruction of the mandible. Plast Reconstr Surg 2014;134(4):628e–34e.

39. van Gemert JT, van Es RJ, Rosenberg AJ, et al. Free vascularized flaps for reconstruction of the mandible: complications, success, and dental rehabilitation. J Oral Maxillofac Surg 2012;70(7):1692–8.

40. Iizuka T, Hafliger J, Seto I, et al. Oral rehabilitation after mandibular reconstruction using an osteocutaneous fibula free flap with endosseous implants. Factors affecting the functional outcome in patients with oral cancer. Clin Oral Implants Res 2005;16(1):69–79.

Surgical Navigation for Oral and Maxillofacial Surgery

Nagi Demian, DDS, MD*, Craig Pearl, DDS,
Timothy Charles Woernley III, DDS, James Wilson, DDS,
Justin Seaman, DDS, MD

KEYWORDS

- Navigation • Minimally invasive surgery • Virtual surgical planning

KEY POINTS

- The applications of navigation technology in oral and maxillofacial surgery continue to increase.
- Navigation involves the use of a preoperative 3-dimensional image, such as a computed tomographic scan, a signal emitter, and a receiver, to provide real-time, precise, and accurate position and guidance during surgery.
- Navigation does not require intraoperative exposure to radiation.
- The integration of virtual surgical planning and navigation technology may decrease operating room time while enhancing surgical accuracy in this new era of patient-specific medicine and surgery.

INTRODUCTION

Surgical navigation has evolved from a stereotactic technique that initially required a frame to a now frameless and more accurate surgical positioning device that provides real-time feedback.

BIOLOGICAL BASIS

Navigation allows surgeons to maneuver through the surgical field with confidence and to place instruments and implants onto the desired location with accuracy and precision. This advantage has been shown to reduce the incidence of repeat procedures.[1] Surgical navigation systems for facial reconstruction rely on accurate imaging (MRI or computed tomography [CT]), a signal emitter, a receiver, and software to interpret the signals. Reference points and emitters vary by application when used with soft or hard tissue. Several steps exist when preparing the system for use and include preoperative imaging, patient and hardware positioning, registration, and verification. After the system is calibrated, surgical navigation allows enhancement of both surgical precision and accuracy owing to real-time confirmation of position, without the need to obtain additional intraoperative images, which expose patients to additional radiation.[2] This is especially important in areas associated with difficult and limited exposure, such as the orbit and deep spaces of the head and neck. When applied to fracture reductions or resection of bony masses, the accuracy of the planned movements or amount of bone removed can be readily measured and palpated. Navigation technology may also facilitate surgery when dealing with soft tissue lesions where access is limited by allowing for minimally invasive access compared with traditional open approaches, which may require extensive dissection for exposure. In addition to such advantages provided in

Disclosure Statement: The authors have nothing to disclose.
Department of Oral and Maxillofacial Surgery, The University of Texas Health Science Center at Houston, 6431 Fannin, Suite JJL 454, Houston, TX 77054, USA
* Corresponding author.
E-mail address: Nagi.demian@uth.tmc.edu

Oral Maxillofacial Surg Clin N Am 31 (2019) 531–538
https://doi.org/10.1016/j.coms.2019.06.001
1042-3699/19/© 2019 Elsevier Inc. All rights reserved.

bone and soft tissue surgery, navigation can be extremely helpful when used for locating and retrieving foreign bodies.

APPLICATION TO ORAL MAXILLOFACIAL SURGERY

The craniomaxillofacial region creates many challenges for the oral and maxillofacial (OMF) surgeon because of the intricate 3-dimensional anatomy, multiple surrounding nerves, and the need for symmetry in the skull. Indications for surgical navigation in OMF surgery have been described as complex unilateral orbital wall fractures comminuted unilateral fractures of the lateral midface, bony tumors, bony reconstruction of complex 3-dimensional anatomy, and for removal of foreign bodies.[3] Furthermore, surgical navigation may be used independently or integrated with VSP software. In an integrated system, the surgeon can place implants or reduce/mirror fractures and compare the intraoperative position to the virtually created plan in real time. For example, in a severely displaced or comminuted unilateral fracture of the mandible or midface, the proper position and orientation of the fractured bone using a mirror image of the uninjured side are planned using VSP. Navigation is then used to verify the reduction of the fractured bone and compare its spatial orientation to the mirrored side. This will instantaneously demonstrate proper reduction without the need to obtain a postoperative CT scan and without additional radiation exposure to the patient. Such utility, as shown by Kim and colleagues,[4] showed a less than 2 mm discrepancy in 36 patients with multiple facial fractures treated with virtual surgical planning and surgical navigation. When integrated with VSP, intraoperative navigation is therefore superior to intraoperative

CT scanning for the evaluation of proper fracture reduction or implant positioning.

EQUIPMENT SETUP

The main components to surgical navigation are the navigation system with attached monitor, a tracker, and an emitter. The navigation system software uses a preoperative CT or MRI image as a map (**Fig. 1**). A tracker is attached to the patient that is then picked up by an emitter (**Fig. 2**). This allows the patient's spatial position to be registered to the navigation system via drawing of specific designs over the patient's face or by touching certain landmarks on the patient's face with the navigation probe. Once the position of the patient is registered and calibrated to the preoperative image displayed on the system screen, navigation can start. Intraoperative accuracy of navigation can be assessed by selecting random soft or hard tissue structures with the probe and comparing its location with the displayed location on the navigation screen.

For the OMF surgeon, additional steps are needed to prevent error in navigation when working on or around the mandible. This is because the additional challenge with registration and verification owing to the mandible being a mobile structure. The position of the mandible at the time of surgery must replicate its position at time of CT acquisition. This is further explained in the case of a foreign body removal presented in later discussion.

CASES
The Orbit

One area where navigation can be quite helpful is the repair of internal orbital fractures. This is due to the small access and the inability to fully expose

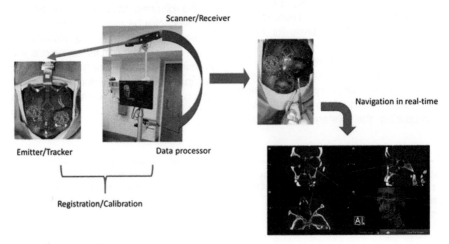

Fig. 1. Overview of a navigation system.

A

B

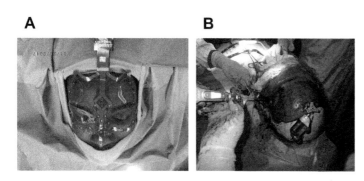

Fig. 2. (A) Skin-borne tracker. (B) Bone-borne tracker.

all aspects of the injury at the same time. Visualization of the fracture is limited, making the repair challenging. If the posterior or medial edges extend far posteriorly, blind instrumentation and placement of hardware can lead to complications, such as damage to the optic nerve or severing of the rectus muscles. Navigation can guide the surgeon during exploration of an orbital fracture and direct the proper placement of an orbital implant.[5]

An example of using navigation for the repair of orbital fractures is shown in **Fig. 3**. The patient presents with diplopia and enophthalmos and reports an antecedent orbital floor fracture that was repaired 3 months before. No intraoperative or postoperative images from his initial injury were available. A CT scan was obtained and showed an inadequate placement of the orbital implant causing an increase in orbital volume. The previously placed implant was removed,

and a new implant was properly placed using surgical navigation during dissection and implant positioning. The final position of the implant was verified using intraoperative CT imaging. Symptoms improved, and no further surgical intervention was required.

Establishment of Bony Contour in Comminuted and Highly Displaced Fractures

Another challenge facing surgeons is the reestablishment of proper reduction and orientation of displaced or comminuted fractured segments. The surgeon can use navigation in the most basic fashion by plotting a point in space to which the fractured bone segment would be brought to. The bony fragment is then mobilized to that point and checked intraoperatively using the navigation probe.

A

B

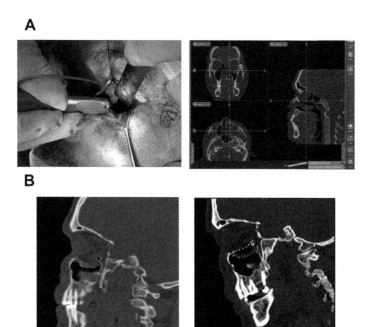

Fig. 3. (A) Navigation for correction of a previously repaired orbital fracture with persisting enophthalmos and diplopia. (B) Preoperative plate clearly maladapted to the posterior edge of the fracture noted in the left photograph. Left photograph shows the postoperative plate position.

In the example shown in **Fig. 4**, a navigation system was used to plot points to reduce a posteriorly displaced zygomaticomaxillary complex (ZMC) fracture. The distances from the malar prominence in the anteroposterior and lateral dimensions were measured on the noninjured side. Comparative points replicating such distances were plotted on the injured side to compensate for the deficiency. The final position was then verified intraoperatively using the navigation probe on the malar bone once in the ideal position.

In the example case shown in **Fig. 5**, a highly comminuted orbitozygomatic fracture was treated in a similar fashion as described by Morrison and colleagues.[6] Using VSP, the projected contour and position of the reduced zygoma were made based on a mirror image of the uninjured side. This was then imported into the navigation system to serve as a guide during reduction and fixation. The accuracy of mirroring for treatment of midface fractures with surgical navigation was found to be predictable despite multiple areas of possible error.[7] Instead of mirroring the uninjured side, stereolithography (STL) files of stock implants can also be used in a similar fashion to guide and reduce the fractured segments and obtain symmetry.

Deep Lesions and Abscesses

Surgical navigation can also be used for the excision or sampling of lesions that are hard to reach without extensive surgical exposure. Such lesions typically involve the posterior maxilla, the base of skull, intracranial structures, or the deep masticator spaces.

Not only can navigation pinpoint the center of such lesions but also can define their perimeter and degree of extension. For deep brain lesions, a bone-borne frame stereotactic navigation system has traditionally been used. Such patients would have a frame fixated to the skull and then undergo a CT study of the same area. This setup allows the surgeon to determine the 3-dimensional position of the lesion based on measurements made to the reference frame. The surgeon may then specifically target the area of the lesion. More contemporary navigation systems are frameless and do not require the additional steps associated with fixation of the frame to the skull.

In the example shown in **Fig. 6**, a deep temporal space infection was unsuccessfully treated with multiple incision and drainage attempts. This was due to a collection posterior to the zygoma that was difficult to drain without an extensive exposure. Furthermore, the infection extended into the orbit via the inferior orbital fissure, causing ophthalmoplegia and severe chemosis. A frameless surgical navigation system was used to reach the collection without increasing surgical exposure while minimizing risk of iatrogenic injury to the posterior orbit. Proper placement of drains was also confirmed in real time. The patient recovered well without vision loss or requirements of additional surgery.

Foreign Bodies

Removal of foreign bodies imbedded in the OMF region may require exploration of critical areas.

A

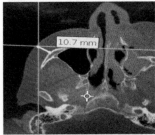
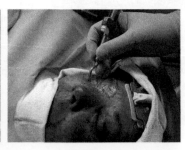

B

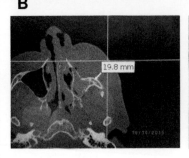
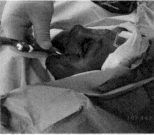

Fig. 4. (A) Use of a navigation probe as a measuring device is a simple method to assist in reestablishing contour of a ZMC fracture. Measuring the distance between the malar prominence on the intact side to the intersection of a line that is perpendicular to the sagittal plane and another perpendicular to the coronal plane crossing the condylar head. (B) Performing the same measurements on the injured side to establish a measured deficit for correction.

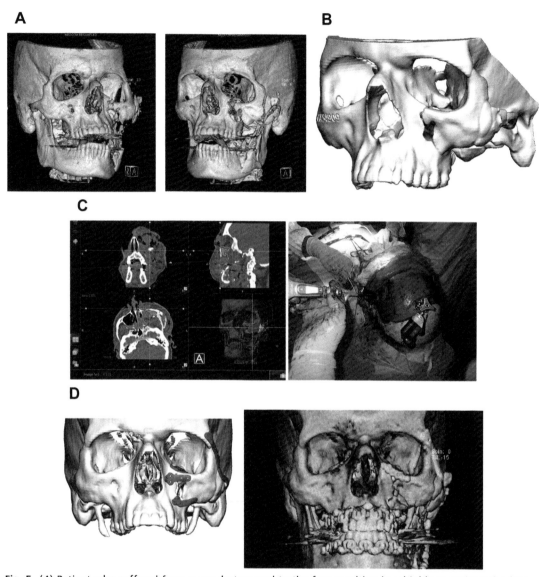

Fig. 5. (*A*) Patient who suffered from a gunshot wound to the face resulting in a highly comminuted orbitozygomatic fracture. (*B*) VSP completed using mirror image from intact side. (*C*) Navigating with VSP plan and uploaded STL data. Note the bone-borne emitter and probe. (*D*) Planned versus actual outcome.

Navigation can precisely locate such foreign body, which limits the need for wide surgical exposure, reduces morbidity, and shortens the surgical time.[8,9] A common scenario encountered by OMF surgeons is a lost needle that fractured during the delivery of local anesthetic for a dental procedure (**Fig. 7**).

When locating a foreign object in the lower facial third, an important additional step to ensure accuracy and precision is required. This is because the mandible is a mobile bone, and therefore, when navigating to locate a foreign object, the same conditions that existed when the CT scan was taken must be duplicated. For example, if a bite block is used while obtaining the CT scan, then the same bite block should be used during surgery to ensure the mouth is open to the same degree. Failure to do so will result in significant errors. The examples in **Figs. 8** and **9** illustrate the advantage of using navigation to locate a foreign object. The patient suffered from a gunshot wound to the mandible years before his presentation. He underwent multiple failed attempts to repair the fracture, resulting in multiple subsequent infections. Navigation allowed for a less invasive approach for the removal the infected bullet fragments in a distorted surgical field secondary to scarring.

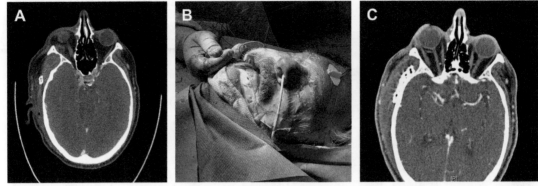

Fig. 6. (*A*) Persistent deep temporal abscess with spread into the orbit via the inferior fissure area. (*B*) Navigation probe used to help locate missed loculation. (*C*) Postoperative CT showing the new drain position.

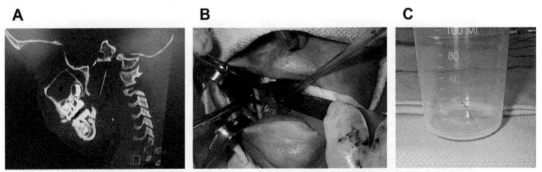

Fig. 7. (*A*) Broken 30-gauge needle in a 6-year-old patient after multiple failed retrieval attempts in a private office. (*B*) Intraoral surgical approach using navigation for a difficult albeit successful retrieval. (*C*) Needle recovered.

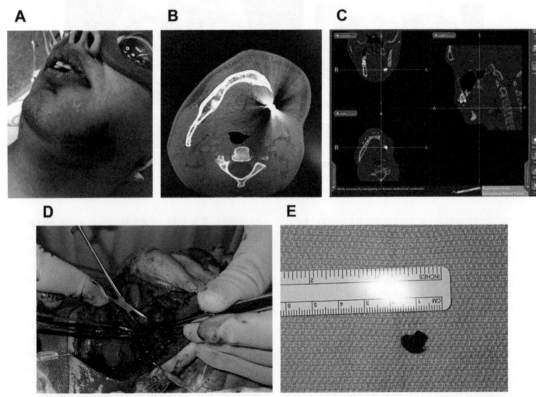

Fig. 8. (*A*) Patient who has suffered a previous gunshot wound to the mandible presents with a recurrent infection, osteocutaneous fistula, and a bony gap. (*B*) Residual bullet fragment after multiple failed retrieval attempts. (*C*) The navigation screen view after upload and registration. (*D*) Locating the fragment with the navigation probe. (*E*) Retrieved bullet fragment.

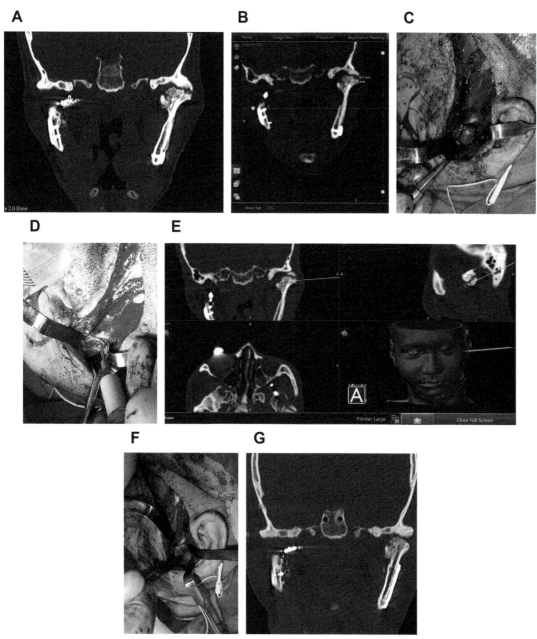

Fig. 9. (*A*) Right temporomandibular ankylosis after suffering extensive facial fractures due to a fall. (*B*) View of the navigation screen after upload and registration. (*C*) Using the navigation probe to assist in locating and resecting/removing the ankylotic mass. (*D*) Outline of ankylotic mass using the navigation system. (*E*) Rotary instrument used to remove ankylotic mass. (*F*) Mobilization of the condyle in preparation for gap arthroplasty. (*G*) Postoperative CT scan.

SUMMARY

Surgical navigation has been shown to be beneficial to the specialty of the OMF surgery. Significant advantages of this modality have been noted for the following cases: complex unilateral orbital wall fractures, comminuted unilateral fractures of the lateral midface, bony tumors, bony reconstruction of complex 3-dimensional anatomy, and for removal of foreign bodies. Despite being a relatively new technology in OMF surgery and the high costs associated with its use, navigation is a tool that has been shown to improve surgical outcomes and reduce operating time. In addition, it has been shown to reduce radiation exposure to patients and the frequency of costly reoperations.

As with all sophisticated technology, there is a steep learning curve. This is especially true for procedures involving the lower third of the face because the mandible is mobile, creating the potential for an error in accuracy. To date, only a few well-scrutinized, randomized, and blinded studies evaluated the cost and time improvements associated with the use of surgical navigation in OMF surgery. At this time, only extrapolation from studies in other disciplines are available, all of which are encouraging.

REFERENCES

1. Bell RB. Computer planning and intraoperative navigation in cranio-maxillofacial surgery. Oral Maxillofac Surg Clin North Am 2010;22(1):135–56.

2. Azarmehr I, Stokbro K, Bell RB, et al. Surgical navigation: a systematic review of indications, treatments, and outcomes in oral and maxillofacial surgery. J Oral Maxillofac Surg 2017;75(9):1987–2005.

3. Lubbers HT, Jacobsen C, Matthews F, et al. Surgical navigation in craniomaxillofacial surgery: expensive toy or useful tool? A classification of different indications. J Oral Maxillofac Surg 2011;69(1):300–8.

4. Kim JW, Wu J, Shen SG, et al. Interdisciplinary surgical management of multiple facial fractures with image-guided navigation. J Oral Maxillofac Surg 2015;73(9):1767–77.

5. Shin HS, Kim SY, Cha HG, et al. Real time navigation-assisted orbital wall reconstruction in blowout fractures. J Craniofac Surg 2016;27(2):370–3.

6. Morrison CS, Taylor HO, Sullivan SR. Utilization of intraoperative 3D navigation for delayed reconstruction of orbitozygomatic complex fractures. J Craniofac Surg 2013;24(3):e284–6.

7. Pierrefeu A, Terzic A, Volz A, et al. How accurate is the treatment of midfacial fractures by a specific navigation system integrating "mirroring" computational planning? Beyond mere average difference analysis. J Oral Maxillofac Surg 2015;73(2):315.e1-10.

8. Xing L, Duan Y, Zhu F, et al. Computed tomography navigation combined with endoscope guidance for the removal of projectiles in the maxillofacial area: a study of 24 patients. Int J Oral Maxillofac Surg 2015;44(3):322–8.

9. Yang CY, Yang RT, He SG, et al. Removal of a large number of foreign bodies in the maxillofacial region with navigation system. Dent Traumatol 2017;33(3):230–4.

Dynamic Navigation for Dental Implant Surgery

Neeraj Panchal, DDS, MD, MA[a],*, Laith Mahmood, DDS, MD[b], Armando Retana, DDS, MD[c], Robert Emery III, DDS[c]

KEYWORDS

- Dental implant navigation • Dental implant surgery • Dental navigation
- Cone-beam computer tomography

KEY POINTS

- Many of the complications associated with the placement of dental implants can be directly related to inaccurate positioning.
- Implant placement using static guided surgery is very accurate; however, it is possible, due to cone-beam computer tomography (CBCT) discrepancy and/or incorrect placement of the guide, for gross deviations in implant position to occur.
- The current dynamic navigation workflow requires (1) a CBCT with fiducials, (2) virtual implant planning, (3) calibration, and (4) implant placement in accordance to the 3-D image on the navigation screen.
- Implant surgeons are able to evaluate a patient, scan the patient, plan the implant position, and perform the implant surgery in the same day without the delay or cost of fabrication of a static surgical guide stent.

INTRODUCTION

Implantologists have several options when it comes to implant planning and placement. Dental implant treatment planning and placement has benefited from accelerating technological capability in office-based imaging and complex simulation and planning software. The combination of software and imaging allowed for the development of static implant guides to achieve predictable accuracy in implant placement. Dynamic navigation (DN) has improved the process by providing surgeons a real-time navigation tool to improve the accuracy of implant placement.

Currently, DN is used by many medical specialties, including ophthalmology, otolaryngology, orthopedics, vascular surgery, neurosurgery, and surgical oncology. These specialties routinely use DN to perform simple and complex procedures with increased accuracy and precision.[1,2] In the field of dentistry, DN historically has been used primarily by oral and maxillofacial surgeons in the hospital. The medical DN systems used were designed primarily for craniomaxillofacial-based procedures, such as orthognathic, trauma, pathology reconstructive procedures and locating foreign bodies within the head and neck.[3,4] In the United States, a DN system was introduced in 2000 to assist in the placement of dental implants in the outpatient office setting. Subsequently, additional systems have been approved for this indication. The current DN workflow requires (1)

Disclosure Statement: The authors have nothing to disclose.
[a] University of Pennsylvania School of Dental Medicine, Penn Presbyterian Medical Center, Philadelphia Veterans Affairs Medical Center, 5 Wright Saunders, 51 North 39th Street, Suite WS-565, Philadelphia, PA 19104, USA; [b] Private Practice, Parkway Oral Surgery and Dental Implant Center, 915 Gessner, Suite 690, Houston, TX 77024, USA; [c] Private Practice, Capital Center for Oral and Maxillofacial Surgery, 2311 M Street Northwest, Suite 200, Washington, DC 20037, USA
* Corresponding author.
E-mail address: npanchal@upenn.edu

Oral Maxillofacial Surg Clin N Am 31 (2019) 539–547
https://doi.org/10.1016/j.coms.2019.08.001

obtaining a three-dimensional (3-D) scan with rigidly fixed or predictably reproducible and accurate fiducial marking systems; (2) virtual implant planning; (3) calibration and registration of fiducial markers, implant drill, and drill lengths with attached tracking arrays; and (4) implant osteotomy and placement in accordance to the 3-D image on the navigation screen.

FREEHANDED APPROACH

Currently, a majority of dental implants are placed freehand, without any form of computer 3-D planning. The surgeon creates an osteotomy using only adjacent and opposing teeth as a reference for position, and places the implant freehanded. When placing multiple implants to restore multiple missing adjacent teeth, a caliper or periodontal probe often is used to ensure appropriate spacing of the implants in a mesiodistal dimension. Intraoperative radiographs may or may not be taken to evaluate the osteotomy and implant position. The most important factor, however, is the clinical emergence of the implant in a restorable position. Position and angulation can be estimated with the use of direction indicators, but the final position must be evaluated at the time of placement by the surgeon. Many of the complications associated with the placement of dental implants can be related directly to inaccurate positioning. These include the following:

- Damage to the inferior alveolar nerve
- Floor of mouth hematoma
- Damage to adjacent roots
- Sinus infections secondary to inadvertent sinus perforations
- Fractured implants due to off-axis loading
- Periimplantitis due to food impaction and off-axis loading
- Poor esthetics secondary to thin buccal, labial bone, and soft tissue
- Interproximal bone loss secondary to placing implants to close to adjacent teeth and implants.
- Increased prosthetic complexity and cost

The intraoperative decision making, predictability, and difficulty in visualizing ideal position and angulation with a freehand approach have steered dentists toward the use of more advanced techniques in implant planning and placement.

STATIC GUIDED APPROACH

In order to aid in position and angulation, multiple types of surgical guides can be used. The most basic type is a stone cast-based static surgical guide. Cast-based surgical implant guides aid in ensuring appropriate restorable position of the implant but do not take into consideration the bone morphology. Further advancement with computer-guided implant surgery, also referred to as guided surgery or static navigation, uses computer-aided design and computer-aided manufacturing surgical templates based on digital planning of implant position, taking into consideration both the restoration and the bony anatomy, on specialized planning software.[5] Several factors have been identified in influencing the accuracy of implants placed using guided surgery. Cone-beam computed tomography (CBCT) precision, model matching to CBCT file, guide fabrication accuracy, guide sleeve tolerance, tissue support of the guide, accurate seating of the guide, patient maximum opening, fully or semiguided technique, and operator experience have all been cited[5–11] Implants placed using a guided approach show less deviation and more predictability than freehand placement, even for experienced surgeons.[9] There also are several clinical scenarios where a static guided surgery may be challenging or not possible, such as a patient with a narrow maximum opening that does not allow for the use of the guide and longer implant drills or limited interdental distance that does not allow for fitting of guide tubes. Although on average, implant placement using static guided surgery is very accurate, it is possible, due to CBCT discrepancy and/or incorrect placement of the guide, for gross deviations in position to occur.

DYNAMIC NAVIGATION TECHNOLOGY

The DN systems available in the United States are a form of computer-assisted surgery (CAS) that use optical tracking. There are 2 types of optical motion tracking systems: active and passive. Active tracking system arrays emit infrared light that is tracked to stereo cameras, and passive tracking system arrays use reflective spheres to reflect infrared light emitted from a light source back to a camera. The patient and drill must be over the line of sight of the tracking camera[12] (**Fig. 1**).

The current most commonly utilized DN technology is passive. Light is projected from a light-emitting diode light source above the patient. The light is projected down to the patient and the surgical field. The light is reflected off tracking arrays (passive patterned arrays) attached to the patient and the surgical instrument being tracked. The reflected light is captured by a pair of stereo cameras above the patient. The DN system then calculates the position of the patient and the

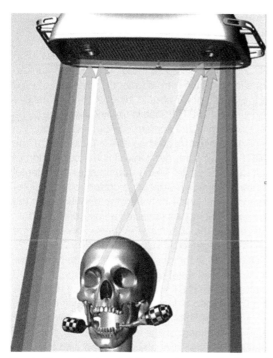

Fig. 1. The patient and drill must be over the line of sight of the tracking camera. (*Courtesy of* X-Nav Technologies, Lansdale, Pennsylvania.)

instruments relative to the presurgical plan. This is done real-time, or dynamically. A virtual image is then projected onto a monitor for the surgeon and staff. This virtual reality device allows the surgeon to work dynamically on the patient and execute the planned implant surgery. At any time, the surgeon can change the plan based on the clinical situation.[13]

DENTATE PATIENT FIDUCIAL

In the dentate patient, the fiducial clip allows for an impression of a patient's teeth to be taken (**Fig. 2**). This impression ensures that the fiducial clip is firmly supported by teeth and the fiducial clip goes into the same location in the patient's mouth every single time when being seated. It is important that the computer tomography (CT) scan is taken with the fiducial clip seated properly in the patient's mouth without any movement or rocking of the fiducial clip. The tracker arm attachment section of the fiducial clip should be on the buccal or cheek side of the patient. The fiducial clip must be placed on the arch where the surgeon is placing the implants but does not interfere with the drilling of the implants. In addition, it should be placed to minimize optical interference by the surgeons or assistants' hands and instruments. Teeth that are mobile, serve as pontics on a bridge, or have orthodontics wires should be avoided.

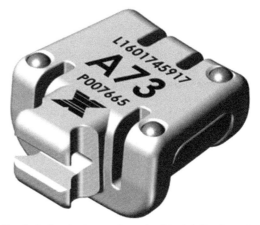

Fig. 2. In the dentate patient, the fiducial clip allows for an impression of the patient's teeth to be taken. (*Courtesy of* X-Nav Technologies, Lansdale, Pennsylvania.)

The fiducial clip is placed in a hot water bath at a temperature of 140°F to 160°F (60°C–71°C) for approximately 3 minutes to 5 minutes. When the thermoplastic on the fiducial clip is clear, it is ready to be used. The fiducial clip should cool for approximately 1 minute to reach a surface temperature less than 104°F (40°C). The fiducial clip is placed on 3 teeth, ensuring an equal distance on the buccal and lingual sides, with the tracker arm positioned on the buccal side. Vertical pressure is applied until the plastic surface cannot go further. Once an adequate impression is taken, the fiducial clip is removed without any rocking motion and then placed in a cold water bath. The fiducial clip then is tried again in the patient's mouth for confirmation of accuracy and to ensure there is no impingement of soft tissue. The fiducial clip should not have any mobility when seated. If there are short clinical crowns or teeth without undercuts, composite can be added to the buccal and occlusal surfaces of the associated teeth to help create immobile fiducial clip insertion. If multiple fiducial clips are placed in the mouth for a dual arch case or additional accuracy, the surgeon must ensure the fiducial clips do not touch.

EDENTULOUS PATIENT FIDUCIAL

An edentulous patient case requires edentulous fiducials (small screws) to be placed in the patient's bone to facilitate registration in the CT scan. The fiducials can be placed through the soft tissue of the patient via small stab incisions apical to the mucogingival junction or directly into the exposed bone by laying a flap. The surgeon must use careful discretion when deciding the location of the edentulous fiducials. The edentulous fiducials are also used in the preoperative process to register with the software prior to surgery. When placing the edentulous fiducials in the mandible, short 4-mm screws should be placed to avoid damage to the inferior alveolar nerve. The screws should be 1.5 mm in diameter, 4 mm or 5 mm in length, self-drilling, self-tapping, low profile, and stable. Typically, a 4-mm screw is recommended in the posterior mandible or in areas of dense cortical bone and 5-mm or greater screws in the maxilla or regions of immature, soft grafted bone. The edentulous fiducials must be placed in the arch where implants will be placed. If implants are to be placed in both the maxilla and the mandible, then edentulous fiducials must be placed in both arches. If vertical bone reduction is anticipated, the edentulous fiducials must be placed apical to the area of proposed bone reduction. The inferior alveolar nerve and the infraorbital nerve must be considered and avoided when placing fiducials. A minimum of 4 fiducials should be placed and spread out throughout the arch, leaving room for an edentulous fiducial plate (**Fig. 3**) to be inserted at the time of surgery.

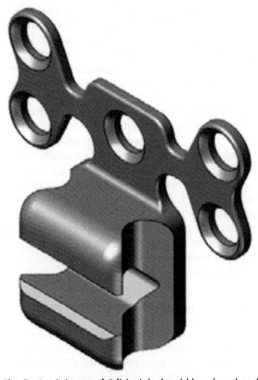

Fig. 3. A minimum of 4 fiducials should be placed and spread out throughout the arch, leaving room for an edentulous fiducial plate to be inserted at the time of surgery. (*Courtesy of* X-Nav Technologies, Lansdale, Pennsylvania.)

IMAGE ACQUISITION AND SOFTWARE PLANNING

Image acquisition includes obtaining 3-D files, usually a CBCT in a Digital Imaging and Communications in Medicine format (.dicom). The field of view of the CBCT or CT should include the surgical site and all fiducials. The scan is obtained with the plane of occlusion of the implant site parallel to floor. An important point related to the acquisition of the CBCT that is often overlooked is the separation of soft tissues while taking the image. For dental implant planning purposes, a cotton roll or radiolucent material place between the dentition and the buccal/labial mucosa creates an air contrast zone. This allows the soft tissue in the region of the free gingival margin to be visualized on the CBCT.

Dual scan is the term used when a dental appliance, such as a set of dentures, is superimposed over a patient's CT scan. If a dual scan technique is utilized, then at least five 2-mm fiducials should be applied to the denture. A high-resolution CT scan is obtained of the denture on its own and then a separate CT scan is obtained with the denture in the patient's mouth, ensuring not to disturb the fiducials on the patient and on the denture.

Another alternative is the use of an intraoral scanner (IOS). An IOS provides a 3-D surface image of the patients' dentition and occlusion. These are not volumetric images; IOS images are a surface. IOS images have a high degree of accuracy for single and quadrant impressions. When full arches are scanned, the accuracy decreases.[8] The implant team may wish to obtain IOS of the patient before teeth are extracted. If the occlusion is not going to be changed, these images can be saved for later use for planning of ideal implant position and provisional fabrication.

Once the images are acquired and stored, they are loaded into treatment planning software. There are numerous software packages available, but some key features should be present related to image processing and analysis. The software should be able to import and export generic file formats (.dicom and .stl), superimpose the 3-D files, perform dual scan .dicom superimposition and be able to export the images in a common coordinate system as an individual or merged item. When these clean .stl images are superimposed on the CBCT data, the combined images allow the implant team to plan, with the osseous, dental, and soft tissue structures clearly visible along with the patient's occlusion.

When starting to plan on the DN software, a panoramic curve for the arch requiring implants is developed on the axial plane of the patient's scan. On the mandible, the inferior alveolar nerve also can be identified and marked. Merger of the patient's scan and the IOS image or denture scan is performed, ensuring there are multiple area of coordination between the images for accuracy of the merger.

The planning of implants should be restoratively driven. This starts with evaluating the occlusion and placing the restorative envelope of the virtual teeth in the proper occlusal position. This can be done using virtual implant crowns available in the DN software. Another option is to use a separate prosthetic software to plan the restorations. The plan is then exported from the prosthetic software and imported as a .stl file into the DN software. Once the implant crown is finalized, the virtual implants should be properly aligned below the virtual crowns for ideal emergence into the prosthetic space. The DN software allows design of a generic implant or previously specified implant, implant platform diameter, implant apex diameter, implant length, and abutment height and angle (**Fig. 4**). Additional tools in the DN software allow mirroring to align implants across an arch and paralleling of adjacent implants.

Calibration

The instruments to be tracked by the system during surgery must be calibrated. The geometry of the tracking arrays relative to the instrument being used must be determined by the tracking system.

The assembled parts must be placed in front of the stereo cameras so the software can "learn" their geometry. The instruments to be calibrated include the contra-angle handpiece, straight handpiece and probe tool.

Registration

The DN system must also be "taught" the geometry of the patient tracking array relative to the fiducials and thus the planned implants. This process is called registration. There is a specific registration workflow for both the dentate and the edentulous patient.

Workflow

The user may select a contra-angle handpiece, probe tool, and straight handpiece. At a minimum, the user must select a handpiece. The workflow adjusts to allow for calibration of the selected items. The calibration of the instrumentation occurs approximately 60 cm to 80 cm from the camera. The contra-angle handpiece along with the handpiece tracker is assembled and calibrated (**Fig. 5**). The handpiece is rotated such that the camera can locate and identify the patterns on the handpiece tracker. After calibration of the handpiece, there is a contra-angle handpiece chuck calibration (**Fig. 6**). The handpiece is attached to the chuck and then the drill motor is

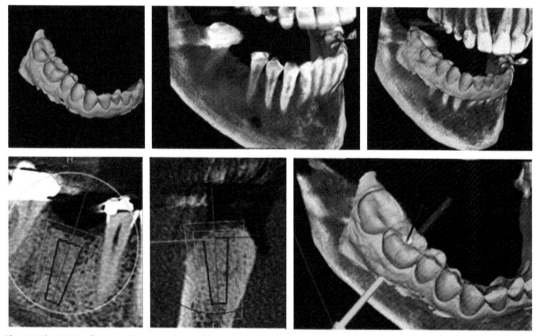

Fig. 4. The DN software allows design of a generic implant or previously specified implant, implant platform diameter, implant apex diameter, implant length, and abutment height and angle.

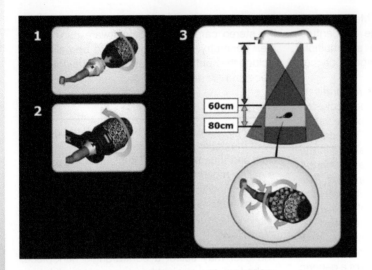

Fig. 5. The contra-angle handpiece along with the handpiece tracker is assembled and calibrated. (*Courtesy of* X-Nav Technologies, Lansdale, Pennsylvania.)

run at 10 to 20 revolutions per minute over the camera to calibrate the chuck plate to the handpiece. A Go Plate (X-Nav Technologies, LLC, Lansdale, Pennsylvania) and probe are calibrated by placing the probe in the pivot hole of the Go Plate. An implant drill bit is placed on the handpiece and the implant drill bit is placed on the Go Plate perpendicular to the center target (**Fig. 7**). The drill length is then verified by the DN system. If drill length measurement registration fails, then the handpiece chuck calibration may need to be executed again.

In the edentulous patient, an edentulous patient calibration probe is calibrated (**Fig. 8**). Then, the edentulous tracker plate is placed on the bone of the patient underneath a subperiosteal flap in an area of the bone where there are no edentulous fiducial screws. The tracker plate is attached to a patient tracker arm and patient tracker. The patient tracker and the edentulous fiducial screws are then registered to the DN system by touching the screws (fiducials) with

the probe as the system tracks them. For the dentate patient, the fiducial clip attached to a patient tracker arm and patient tracker is registerd automatically by the system at the time of calibration.

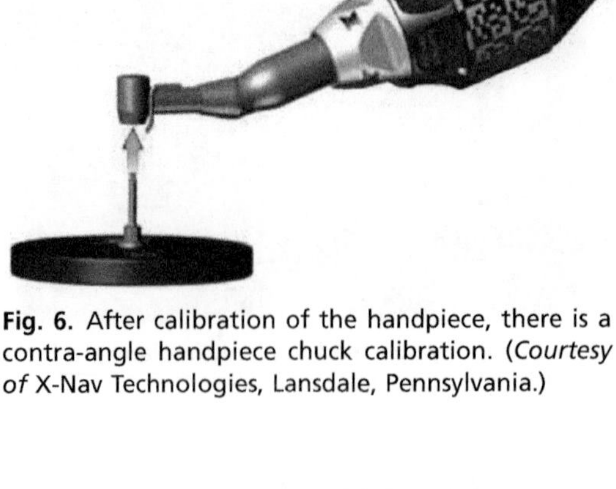

The calibration accuracy is verified between the fiducials and the drill. The drill bit is placed on 3 fiducial spheres on the fiducial clip for the dentate patient or the edentulous fiducial screws. The doctor looks at the two-dimensional (2-D) views for accuracy data in green colors. If all three fiducials have green indicators the system calibration is within 200 micrometers. This step is not performed with edentulous patients.

Prior to the start of surgery and after every drill bit is changed there is a "system check" performed by the doctor. This step ensures the instruments are calibrated and the system is properly registered to the patient.

PERFORMING DYNAMIC NAVIGATION SURGERY

It is important to always confirm the accuracy of the tracking system by performing frequent system checks. Anatomical landmarks on the patient are touched with the instruments. The doctor then visually confirms that the radiographic landmarks on the screen are exactly correlating. The optimal landmarks are adjacent teeth or boney landmarks close to the planned implant site or fiducial markers on edentulous patients. The operator looks at the screen as the drill is positioned over the surgical site. The navigation system screen allows viewing of a virtual drill with demonstration of the depth in tenths of a millimeter, angular deviation of the drill bit axis from the planned implant axis to the tenths of a degree and the implant

Fig. 6. After calibration of the handpiece, there is a contra-angle handpiece chuck calibration. (*Courtesy of* X-Nav Technologies, Lansdale, Pennsylvania.)

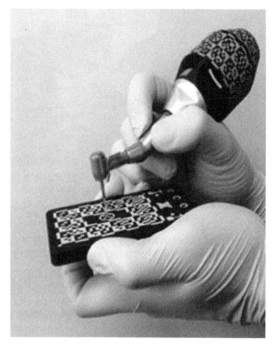

Fig. 7. An implant drill bit is placed on the handpiece and the implant drill bit is place on the Go Plate perpendicular to the center target. (*Courtesy of* X-Nav Technologies, Lansdale, Pennsylvania.)

timing. The tip of the drill, a blue dot, is positioned over the target to indicate ideal planned platform position. The top of the drill a small circle is then centered over the blue dot to indicate ideal planned angle. Depth is indicated by color, yellow, green the red. The planned depth is always at the 45 position on the target. The surgical assistant is in charge of suctioning and looking into the surgical field to notify the surgeon of any irregularities such as lack of irrigation or grossly off-positioned drill placement (**Fig. 9**). As implant drilling occurs,

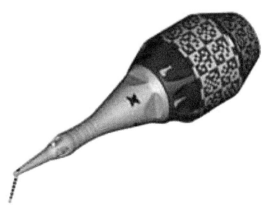

Fig. 8. In the edentulous patient, an edentulous patient calibration probe is calibrated. (*Courtesy of* X-Nav Technologies, Lansdale, Pennsylvania.)

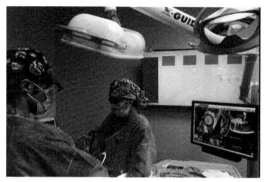

Fig. 9. The surgical assistant is in charge of suctioning and looking into the surgical field to notify the surgeon of any irregularities, such as lack of irrigation or grossly off-positioned drill placement. (*Courtesy of* X-Nav Technologies, Lansdale, Pennsylvania.)

the depth indicator changes in color from green to yellow when the drill is 0.5mm from the targeted depth. The yellow will turn to red indicating when to stop the depth of the osteotomy (**Fig. 10**). During the implant surgery the implant size, width, type and location can be adjusted based on intraoperative factors deemed necessary for a stable and appropriately restorable implant.

DYNAMIC NAVIGATION ADVANTAGES

Implant surgeons are able to evaluate a patient, scan the patient, plan the implant position, and perform the implant surgery in the same day without the delay or cost of fabrication of a static surgical guide stent. This technology also allows the implant surgeon to change the implant size, system, and location parameters intraoperatively when clinical situations dictate a change. DN allows surgeons the confidence to know implant placement is appropriately in bone without having to open a flap, thus minimizing trauma to the patient.

The major benefit of DN is that it allows the surgeon to verify accuracy at all times of the surgery, as opposed to the static technique, where, if the splint is not appropriately positioned and fixated, there can be significant gross error of the entire implant surgery. The inaccurate placement of dental implants placed freehand has been documented in the dental literature.[14–16] There is a mean angular deviation for edentulous mucosal born guides of 2.71° (SD 1.36) versus freehand of 9.92° (SD 6.01). The mean angular deviations are similar for DN placed implants of 2.97° (SD 2.08) compared with freehand of 6.50° (SD 4.21).[16] Any form of CAS is statistically more accurate and precise than freehand placement because it overcomes the inherent inaccuracy of human vision. Crucially, the dynamic approach to implant

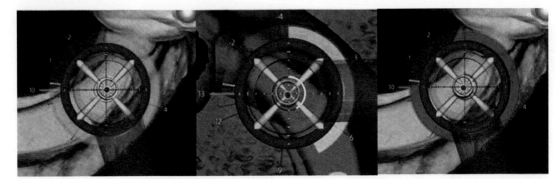

Fig. 10. As implant drilling occurs, the depth indicator changes in color from green to yellow when the drill is 0.5 mm from the targeted depth. The yellow turns to red, indicating when to stop the depth of the osteotomy. (*Courtesy of* X-Nav Technologies, Lansdale, Pennsylvania.)

placement has implant failure rates similar to those of static and traditional approaches.

Ergonomically, DN allows the surgeon to look at the screen more so than inside the mouth, decreasing the need to bend the back or neck for a prolonged period. DN also allows the surgeon to perform the osteotomy and place the implant with limited direct visualization in the mouth in patients with limited mouth opening or in cases of posterior implant placement with difficult visualization. It also allows for guidance of implant placement when interdental spaces prohibit appropriate guidance tubes with static guides, such as in the mandibular incisor region.

DYNAMIC NAVIGATION DISADVANTAGES

The implementation of DN requires significant investment for the dental implant surgeon. In addition to a CBCT and an IOS, there is the capital cost of the DN system. There is also per-case cost of fiducial clips, markers, and plates. Those surgeons with limited experience with technology and virtual image processing may find it difficult to transition to a different modality of practice. There is also a learning curve with the application of a new technology for all levels of technological comfort. The learning curve for one DN system was evaluated. The surgeon become statistically equivalent, proficient, after 10 to 20 implants placed with the system.[15] In addition, restorative dentist will require training to be comfortable with the workflow implemented by the implant surgeon.

Another downside is that the current FDA approved systems for edentulous patients require the additional surgery of the placement of fiducial screws and tracking plates. This obstacle will soon be replaced with a fiducial free method. The patient's anatomy will take the place of the screws. The doctor will select specific points on the CBCT during planning. After the patient tracker

is placed the patient will be registered by toughing those points with the calibrated probe. Both dentate and edentulous patient must have also a potentially cumbersome tracking arms attached to their mouth. As the DN systems hardware and software mature these disadvantage will diminish.

SUMMARY

The natural progression from analog 2-D imaging and diagnostics to digital 3-D imaging and diagnostics has led to increased understanding of the complex nature of implant surgery and prosthetics. The increased utilization of these digital 3-D diagnostic and therapeutic modalities allows the surgical team to see the limitations of freehand surgery. CAS allows the implant team to overcome the limitations of human stereo vision and increase the accuracy and precision of implant placement. DN allows the surgeon to implement digital implant treatment plans in an efficient fashion. This efficiency and flexibility allow the team to utilize CAS on every implant in every patient. High-level statistical evidence clearly illustrates the improved accuracy and precision of CAS over freehand surgery.

REFERENCES

1. Mezger U, Jendrewski C, Bartels M. Navigation in surgery. Langenbecks Arch Surg 2013;398:501–14.
2. Clarke JV, Deakin AH, Nicol AC, et al. Measuring the positional accuracy of computer assisted surgical tracking systems. Comput Aided Surg 2010;15(1–3):13–8.
3. Gerbino G, Zavattero E, Berrone M, et al. Management of needle breakage using intraoperative navigation following inferior alveolar nerve block. J Oral Maxillofac Surg 2013;71:1819.
4. Bobek SL. Applications of navigation for orthognathic surgery. Oral Maxillofac Surg Clin North Am 2014;26:587.

5. Rungcharassaeng K, Caruso JM, Kan JYK, et al. Accuracy of computer-guided surgery: a comparison of operator experience. J Prosthet Dent 2015; 114(3):407–13.

6. Turbush SK, Turkyilmaz I. Accuracy of three different types of stereolithographic surgical guide in implant placement: an in vitro study. J Prosthet Dent 2012; 108(3):181–8.

7. Raico Gallardo YN, da Silva-Olivio IRT, Mukai E, et al. Accuracy comparison of guided surgery for dental implants according to the tissue of support: a systematic review and meta-analysis. Clin Oral Implants Res 2017;28(5):602–12.

8. Kernen F, Benic GI, Payer M, et al. Accuracy of Three-Dimensional Printed Templates for Guided Implant Placement Based on Matching a Surface Scan with CBCT. Clin Implant Dent Relat Res 2016; 18(4):762–8.

9. Vermeulen J. The accuracy of implant placement by experienced surgeons: guided vs freehand approach in a simulated plastic model. Int J Oral Maxillofacial Implants 2017;32(3):617–24.

10. Laederach V, Mukaddam K, Payer M, et al. Deviations of different systems for guided implant surgery. Clin Oral Implants Res 2017;28(9): 1147–51.

11. Cassetta M, Bellardini M. How much does experience in guided implant surgery play a role in accuracy? A randomized controlled pilot study. Int J Oral Maxillofac Surg 2017;46(7):922–30.

12. Strong EB, Rafii A, Holhweg-Majert B, et al. Comparison of 3 optical navigation systems for computer-aided maxillofacial surgery. Arch Otolaryngol Head Neck Surg 2008;134(10):1080–4.

13. Block MS, Emery RW. Static or dynamic navigation for implant placement—choosing the method of guidance. J Oral Maxillofac Surg 2016;74:269.

14. Block MS, Emery RW, Lank K, et al. Implant placement accuracy using dynamic navigation. Int J Oral Maxillofac Implants 2017;32:92.

15. Block MS, Emery RW, Cullum DR, et al. Implant placement is more accurate using dynamic navigation. J Oral Maxillofac Surg 2017;75:1377.

16. Emery RW, Merritt SA, Lank K, et al. Accuracy of dynamic navigation for dental implant placement–model-based evaluation. J Oral Implantol 2016; 42:399.

Evolving Technologies for Tissue Cutting

Jonathon S. Jundt, DDS, MD[a],*, Jose M. Marchena, DMD, MD[a,b], Issa Hanna, DDS[a,c], Jagtar Dhanda, BDS, MFDS RCS(Eng), MBBS, MRCS(Eng), FRCS(OMFS), PhD[d], Matthew J. Breit, DMD[a], Andrew P. Perry, DDS[a]

KEYWORDS

- Ultrasonic surgery • Plasma scalpels • Waterjet surgery
- Rapid evaporative ionization mass spectroscopy (REIMS)

KEY POINTS

- Improved technologies for tissue cutting increase surgical precision, reduce or eliminate thermal injury of adjacent tissues, reduce blood loss, decrease operating time, and may improve outcomes.
- Modern ultrasonic cutting devices reduce the extent of adjacent thermal injury of bone as well as thermal and mechanical injury of surrounding soft tissues compared with traditional rotary instruments or saws.
- Plasma beams used as cutting devices have been shown to cut with equal or more precision compared with conventional blades and generate reduced levels of thermal injury, inflammation, and scarring compared with conventional electrosurgery.
- Waterjet dissection allows for precise dissection and ablation of tissues without generating heat and without causing significant structural injury to nerves and vessels.
- The application of Rapid Ionization Evaporative Mass Spectroscopy of surgical smoke generated by electrocautery is currently undergoing human clinical trials to allow for real-time detection of tumor and assessment of surgical margins.

INTRODUCTION

Surgical manipulation of tissue evolved during the early twentieth century from stainless steel blades and chisels to electric current–powered cauterization, electric handpieces, and saws. Changes resulted from a shift in the type of energy used from human hands to electric current–based power. Manipulation of energy continues to drive advancement in tissue cutting technologies.

The goal of tissue cutting technologies is to divide tissue with precision, limit damage to adjacent tissues, reduce operating time, limit blood loss, and reduce scar tissue. Lasers, ultrasonic devices, plasma beam scalpels, and waterjet scalpels cut tissues with advantages specific to their indications. Bone cutting through ultrasonic methods has increased in popularity, yet rotary and oscillating devices remain the most commonly used modalities. Soft tissue ultrasonic technologies alter tissue through cutting, coaptation, coagulation, or cavitation. Plasma beam scalpels function by adding energy to a gas and demonstrate a high degree of precision and elimination of unintended tissue trauma. Waterjet dissection separates tissues through a focused beam of normal saline instead of burning or fusing.

Disclosure Statement: The authors have nothing to disclose.
[a] Department of Oral and Maxillofacial Surgery, The University of Texas Health Science Center at Houston, 7500 Cambridge Street, Suite 6100, Houston, TX 77054, USA; [b] Ben Taub Hospital, Houston, TX, USA; [c] Lyndon B. Johnson Hospital, Houston, TX, USA; [d] Maxillofacial/Head and Neck Surgery, Queen Victoria Hospital, Holtye Road, East Grinstead RH19 3DZ, UK
* Corresponding author.
E-mail address: jonathon.jundt@uth.tmc.edu

Oral Maxillofacial Surg Clin N Am 31 (2019) 549–559
https://doi.org/10.1016/j.coms.2019.07.009
1042-3699/19/Published by Elsevier Inc.

rapid evaporative ionization mass spectroscopy (REIMS) is an investigational technology that analyzes the surgical smoke vapors for malignant cells to assist in identifying surgical margins in real time.

This section describes the mechanism of action, reviews current literature, and examines clinical indications and potential limitations of evolving and less discussed tissue cutting modalities. Ultrasonic devices, plasma beam scalpels, waterjets, and REIMS are discussed and their applications in oral and maxillofacial surgery reviewed.

ULTRASONIC CUTTING DEVICES
Technology

Ultrasonic technology was initially used by dentists in the 1950s as ultrasonic scalers. It was later applied to tissue cutting devices for ophthalmology, neurosurgery, and general surgery with the development of the phacoemulsifier, cavitational ultrasonic surgical aspirator, and ultrasonic scalpel. Most ultrasonic tissue cutting devices available today are essentially piezoelectric oscillators that produce ultrasonic waves that are transferred to the tissue via a surgical tip. Depending on the frequency of the waves, tissues may be cut, coapted, or coagulated.

Jacques and Pierre Curie discovered the piezoelectric effect in the 1880s.[1] They found that if 2 conducting surfaces applied pressure to certain types of crystals, a potential would cause molecules of the crystal to reorient.[1] It was later found that if alternating currents were applied, back and forth motion of the crystal molecules would generate high-speed vibrations and waves.[2] The energy of such waves can have different effects on tissues when delivered at different frequencies.

The cavitation effect, which is based on Bernoulli's law, is a tissue response to the transduced mechanical waves. According to Bernoulli's law, when a high-speed stream of water is created, the pressure within that stream is so low that the water molecules vaporize causing a collapse of water pockets.[3] This collapse is seen as cavitation or cutting when ultrasonic waves are transferred to tissues. Depending on the frequency and amplitude applied, different types of tissues are cut.[4]

Ultrasonic bone cutting devices rely on the vibration-induced cavitation effect and mechanical pressure exerted on the bone by the device. In order to allow for mineralized tissues to be cut while preserving soft tissues, piezo bone cutting devices use low-frequency vibrations of 60 to 200 m/s at 24 to 29 kHz.[5] Such low-frequency vibrations also reduce the amount of heat generated and may limit unintended tissue damage.[5] Bone

cutting and piezo cutting devices marketed under differing trade names include Piezo Surgical Piezotome Ultrasonic, SurgySonic, Piezon Master Surgery, VarioSurg, Surgybone, Piezosurgery, and Sonopet ultrasonic aspirator.

For soft tissue cutting devices, vibration frequencies are increased to greater than 50 kHz.[6] Soft tissue cutting devices also allow for the processes of coaptation and coagulation. Coaptation refers to the disruption of hydrogen bonds in tissues, causing collagen molecules to collapse and adhere to each other forming a tenacious coaptation during the initial delivery of the energy and early increase in temperature.[3] Coaptation allows for the sealing of vessels while the tissue is being squeezed by the device and aids in the achievement of hemostasis. If energy is applied for a longer period, a further increase in temperature occurs, leading to the release of water and vapor and subsequent coagulation.[3] Currently available ultrasonic devices with these capabilities are sold as Harmonic shears or scalpels.

Excessive heat transfer during bone cutting can lead to undesired bone necrosis, resulting in fracture nonunions, hardware failure, or osteomyelitis. Bone necrosis and impaired cell turnover are seen at temperatures greater than 47 C/116.6 F for at least 1 minute.[7] One advantage of piezo bone cutting devices is that they produce less heat compared with traditional rotary instruments and saws, resulting in a decreased risk for bone and soft tissue necrosis.[7] A tip designed for implant site osteotomies was shown to produce less thermal and mechanical damage to adjacent bone.[4] When comparing a piezo device with a conventional implant drill, Preti and colleagues[8] found greater new bone formation with more osteoblasts during the initial 7 to 10 days along with a decrease in proinflammatory cytokines (**Fig. 1**).

Applications in Oral and Maxillofacial Surgery

Technological improvements in ultrasonic cutting devices have increased their utilization in oral and maxillofacial surgery.[7] Ultrasonic bone cutting applications have been applied to dentoalveolar, orthognathic, craniofacial, and temporomandibular joint surgical procedures. Dentoalveolar procedures include implant site preparation, tooth extraction, bone harvesting, sinus floor access and augmentation, ridge splitting, and lateralization of the inferior alveolar nerve. Multiple animal models have demonstrated greater osteocyte viability and reduced cell death when osteotomies were performed with a piezo ultrasonic device

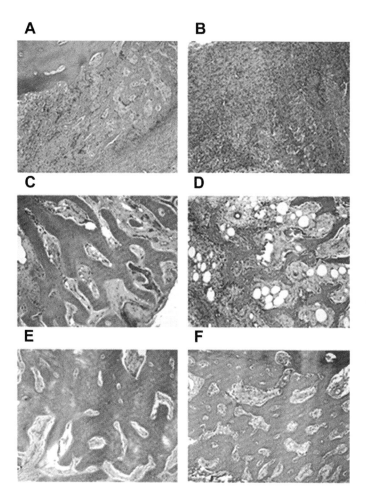

Fig. 1. Postdecalcification histologic sections. Sample obtained at day 7 from the piezoelectric bone surgery site (*B*) shows more newly formed bone and a higher number of osteoblasts than the sample from the drilled site (*A*). A sample obtained at day 14 from a piezoelectric bone surgery site (*D*) shows more newly formed bone and a higher number of osteoblasts than the sample from the drilled site (*C*). Samples obtained at day 56 from drilled (*E*) and piezoelectric bone surgery (*F*) sites show similarly formed bone (hematoxylin and eosin, original magnification × 100). (*Adapted from* Preti G, Martinasso G, Peirone B, et al. Cytokines and growth factors involved in the osseointegration of oral titanium implants positioned using piezoelectric bone surgery versus a drill technique: a pilot study in minipigs. J Periodontol 2007;78:716–22; with permission.)

compared with conventional rotary drills[4] (see **Fig. 1**). Increased preservation of osteogenic potential of the grafts leads to higher graft success rates through limited resorption, enhanced healing, and predictable remodeling. Furthermore, ultrasonic cutting has also been shown to reduce morbidity at the harvest site.[4]

One of the early applications of piezo bone cutting technology in oral surgery was its use in sinus lifting procedures. This has been traditionally carried out with a bur at a high rpm on a surgical handpiece. Generally, a Caldwell-Luc window is created to access the membrane, which is then mechanically elevated using angled curettes. Schneiderian membrane perforations may occur during the lateral osteotomy or during the sinus membrane elevation maneuver. Such perforations have been shown to increase the risk of infection and bone graft loss by 2-fold.[8] The use of a piezo device has been was shown to be associated with a reduced risk of such membrane perforations.[4,9,10] In a meta-analysis comparing piezo versus conventional rotary

instrumentation devices, Jordi and colleagues[10] found that the conventional technique had a 24% rate of perforation versus an 8% rate using the piezo device. Vercellotti and colleagues[11] also reported a low perforation rate of 5% in a case series of 15 patients undergoing open sinus lifting with a piezo device.

Traditional cutting devices used for osteotomies in craniofacial surgery include chisels, reciprocating saws, or burs. Many of these osteotomies are performed in areas adjacent to critical structures such as the dura or orbits, often with limited bone thickness. Piezo cutting devices cut bone at frequencies that are lower than required to cause injury soft tissue, making them safe alternatives for carrying osteotomies with a reduced risk of injury to blood vessels, nerves, and dura.[11] Although cutting times may be longer with the use of a piezo device, total operating time has not been demonstrated to increase.[12,13] During craniofacial advancements in pediatric patients, an 18% decrease in blood loss was shown with ultrasonic bone cutting.[12] When used for osteotomies in orthognathic surgery, ultrasonic cutting tips allow for precise bony cuts with limited injury to adjacent bone or teeth (**Fig. 2**). A decrease in blood loss and a reduced incidence of nerve injury was also shown while cutting with greater accuracy.[14] In addition, Rossi and colleagues[15] also reported decreased postoperative edema and pain in patients undergoing bimaxillary surgery.[16,17]

The advantages provided by the ultrasonic bone cutting devices have also been shown in temporomandibular joint surgery. Temporomandibular joint procedures require precise cuts in proximity to the middle cranial fossa, external auditory canal, and the masseteric and internal maxillary arteries.[18] Silva and colleagues[18] found a 49% reduction in blood loss when using an ultrasonic cutting device for temporomandibular joint surgery compared with a reciprocating saw.

Although mostly used for bone cutting in oral and maxillofacial surgery, ultrasonic surgery is also used for soft tissue dissection. Ultrasonic soft tissue cutting devices are referred to as ultrasonic shears. These devices are primarily used for neck dissections because of their capability to achieve excellent hemostasis with limited collateral thermal injury to adjacent tissues and nerves. Other applications include salivary gland removal and thyroidectomy where collateral thermal injury to adjacent structures such as the facial nerve, recurrent laryngeal nerve, or parathyroid glands can lead to serious adverse outcomes.

Phillips and colleagues[19] compared lateral energy injury to adjacent tissue of 4 commercially available ultrasonic (Harmonic Ace and Harmonic LCS-5) and bipolar devices (Gyrus Trisector and LigaSure V) in a porcine model. They showed that the ultrasonic devices caused the least thermal injury with superficial and full-thickness energy spreads measuring 2.8 mm and 2.4 mm, respectively, compared with bipolar electrosurgical devices.[19] Their results are summarized in **Table 1**. With regard to injury to adjacent nerve tissue, Chen and colleagues[20] compared the effects of electrosurgery versus an ultrasonic device on incisions close to the sciatic nerve in rats. They found that use of the ultrasonic device resulted in a lower frequency of neural impairment and less inflammation.[20] With regard to blood loss, Upadhyaya and colleagues[21] carried out a meta-analysis of hemostasis techniques used in thyroid surgery and found that there was no statistical difference in blood loss when using a bipolar versus an ultrasonic shears. They also showed that they were able to seal vessels of up to 5 mm in diameter with ultrasonic shears and confirmed the effectiveness of the seal under a stimulated systolic pressure of 222 mm Hg.

In summary, the use of ultrasonic cutting technology has allowed oral and maxillofacial surgeons to carry out operations with greater surgical precision, reduced thermal injury to adjacent tissues, decreased blood loss, and improved overall outcomes.

PLASMA CUTTING
Technology

Four fundamental states of matter are known and include solids, liquids, gases, and plasma. Plasma forms when an externally applied heat or a strong electromagnetic field is subjected to an inert gas. Several types of plasma-based cutting devices are currently in use. Earlier applications of plasma in surgery focused on the thermal effects of plasma, yet, the nonthermal effects are of more contemporary interest for potential roles in genetic

A   **B**

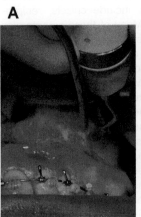 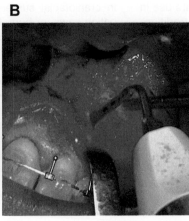

Fig. 2. Segmental LeFort I osteotomy with a piezo ultrasonic cutting tip. (*A*) Precise maxillary wall cut with no visible charring and with minimal bone loss or chipping. (*B*) Thin precise interdental cut minimizing risk for mechanical or thermal injury to the teeth. (*Courtesy of* David Alfi DDS, MD, Houston, TX.)

Table 1
Full-thickness and superficial lateral energy spread (measured in mm) of ultrasonic and electrosurgical soft tissue coagulation and cutting devices

	Harmonic ACE (Mean ± SD) (n)	Harmonic LCS-C5 (Mean ± SD) (n)	Trisector (Mean ± SD) (n)	Ligasure (Mean ± SD) (n)
Overall Full-Thickness Mean	2.4 + 1.3 (29)	3.1 + 1.8 (35)	6.3 + 2.6 (35)	4.5 ± 1.7 (30)
Overall Superficial Mean	2.8 ± 1.3 (29)	4.3 ± 1.8 (35)	7.0 ± 2.7 (32)	5.9 ± 2.6 (30)

Data from Phillips CK, Hruby GW, Durak E, et al. Tissue response to surgical energy devices. Urology 2008;71:744–8; with permission.

transfection, cell detachment, bacterial deactivation, direct plasma-medical sterilization of living tissue, and wound healing with excellent precision and limited effects on surrounding tissues.[22] Nonthermal plasma–assisted blood coagulation mechanisms of action have not been elucidated; however, contemporary theories regarding the coagulative properties suggest direct nonthermal plasma acting directly on blood clotting proteins and promotion of platelet activation.[22] As the oxygen and nitrogen in the ambient air becomes highly charged, reactive particles are formed that have the potential to destroy bacteria and abnormal cells. Although many theoretic advantages of plasma technology are under investigation, several devices are currently available and approved for clinical use. The plasma scalpel was first reported in the journal of Medical Progress through Technology in 1976 by Link, Incropera, and Glover.[23] A 3000-degree Celsius gas jet incised and cauterized tissues with decreased hemorrhage as compared with steel or traditional electrosurgical instruments.[23] Glover and colleagues[24] reported a human trial in 1982 that involved 96 patients representing 138 procedures. The plasma scalpel in this study used argon gas subjected to a direct current arc, which ionized the gas. It was found to effectively divide and coagulate tissue with a shorter time to achieve hemostasis than electrosurgical devices available at that time.[24]

Currently available devices marketed as plasma-based technologies include the PlasmaJet, J-Plasma, Canady Hybrid Plasma, and Plasmablade. Each instrument functions through a proprietary energy waveform coupled with a noble gas, excluding the Plasmablade that functions via an electric arc and ionization of ambient air. Lower temperatures as compared with standard electrosurgical devices is realized across all devices with the benefit of reduced collateral tissue damage, improved hemostasis, and potentially improved healing.

The J-Plasma is a 510K FDA-approved electrosurgical cutting device that uses helium gas molecules excited by an electric field to produce a plasma stream. It also features a retractable blade for manually cutting soft tissue. It is indicated for both open and laparoscopic procedures with the plasma function indicated to coagulate and the blade indicated to cut tissues. Total energy output for the system is 40 Watts (W) of a proprietary radiofrequency waveform through a monopolar delivery system. Advantages of the helium-based plasma cutting technology include minimal thermal spread and damage to adjacent or underlying tissues. Pedroso and colleagues[25] evaluated the lateral spread and depth of thermal spread of monopolar, argon, laser and j-plasma porcine intestine, bladder, and peritoneal tissues at 15% power, 4 L/min gas flow, Bovie monopolar pencil at cut setting of 30 W, Argon Beam Coagulator at 70 W, 4 L/min, and CO_2 laser super pulse at 12 W. It was found that the cold plasma device, J-plasma, achieved comparable and, in some instances, decreased collateral tissue damage during testing. Decreased damage to surrounding tissues also reduces surgical smoke plume and the attendant risks to the practitioner.

Applications in Oral and Maxillofacial Surgery

The J-plasma has several applications in oral and maxillofacial surgery, including cervicoplasty, skin tightening, face lifts, neck dissection, chronic wound care, hypertrophic scarring, and tumor resection.[26] Currently, a clinical trial is underway investigating the use of J-plasma in the reduction of facial rhytides. It is a multicenter, single-arm, evaluator-blind prospective study of 55 subjects seeking to reduce the appearance of wrinkles.[25] The focused beam in comparison to other modalities is illustrated in **Fig. 3**. Cancer treatment applications of cold plasma have demonstrated robust antitumor effects with preliminary results

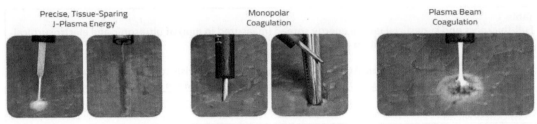

Precise, Tissue-Sparing
J-Plasma Energy

Monopolar
Coagulation

Plasma Beam
Coagulation

Fig. 3. Comparison of J-Plasma, monopolar coagulation, and plasma beam coagulation. (*Courtesy of* Apyx Medical, Purchase, NY.)

implicating deregulation of cell adhesion, cell proliferation, growth regulation, and cell death through development of reactive oxygen species and reactive nitrogen species.[27]

WATERJET CUTTING
Technology

Waterjet cutting, or hydrosurgery, is a technology used for tissue dissection and ablation. Although the technology has existed for many years, applications continue to emerge in various surgical specialties. Waterjet cutting requires the generation of a precise high-velocity waterjet stream. The cutting or ablative effect is a direct result of the erosive forces by the waterjet on the tissues (**Fig. 4**).

The waterjet selectively separates tissues based on their density and mechanical characteristics without thermal injury.[28] Softer tissues such as parenchyma, loose connective, or necrotic tissue are separated and washed away from adjacent nerves and vessels that contain higher proportions of collagen and elastin.[28] Exposed vessels may then be selectively ligated or coagulated with ultrasonic devices, plasma beam, or conventional

electrocautery. Conceptual advantages of waterjet cutting are the controlled preservation of vessels that can cause intraoperative bleeding and the lack of thermal injury to adjacent tissues, particularly nerves (see **Fig. 4**).

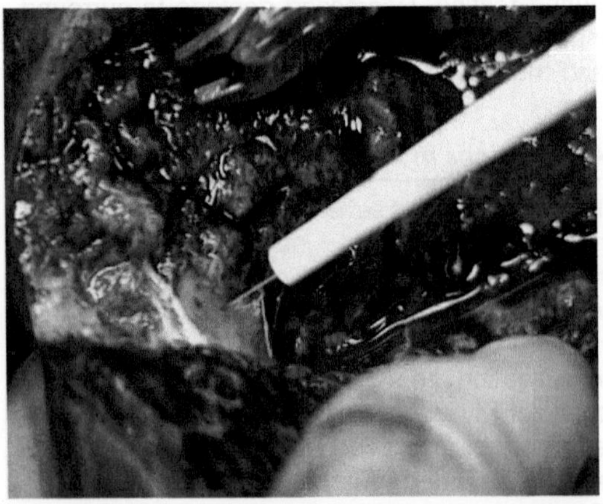

Clinically, waterjets (normal saline) have been predominantly used for liver resection,[29] neurosurgical procedures,[30] prostate ablation,[31–33] and wound debridement.[34] The appropriate waterjet pressure and nozzle size are dictated by the type of tissue and surgical goals. For liver resections, for example, it was shown that although a jet pressure of 30 to 40 bar and nozzle size of 0.1 mm is effective to dissect liver tissue, a pressure of 10 bar higher is needed in cases of an indurated cirrhotic liver.[29] In experimental parotidectomy models in dogs, it was shown that a waterjet pressure of 40 to 60 bar with a nozzle size of 120 microns allowed for atraumatic dissection of the facial nerve with preservation of its function.[35] Similar parameters were described in a report on 10 patients.[36]

One important drawback of using waterjet as a sole method for dissection is the inability to coagulate vessels without changing devices. Recent developments, however, include integration of the waterjet into a hollow coagulation tip as a single device allowing for waterjet dissection and coagulation without changing instruments (**Fig. 5**).

In one such device, waterjet is integrated with a traditional electrosurgical tip.[37] A similar hybrid device is now available by incorporation of waterjet with argon plasma coagulation.[38] Another recent development is the integration of waterjet with image-guided robotic surgery for prostate ablation.[31–33] The emerging data on prostate ablation is particularly important in that it suggests a reduced incidence of sexual dysfunction due to nerve injury compared with traditional methods of prostate ablation.

Applications in Oral and Maxillofacial Surgery

Waterjet surgery has been used for parotidectomy,[36] tonsillectomy,[39] and as facial waterjet-assisted liposuction as an alternative to

Fig. 4. Waterjet cutting of liver parenchyma. Notice the preservation of fine vascular structures and the lack of charring of the cut surfaces. (*Courtesy of* Erbe Elektromedizin GmbH, Tuebingen, Germany.)

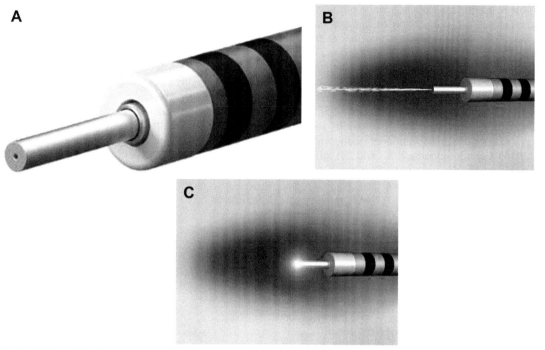

Fig. 5. (*A*) Hybrid knife system showing (*B*) waterjet and (*C*) argon plasma coagulation within the same tip. (*Courtesy of* Erbe Elektromedizin GmbH, Tuebingen, Germany.)

conventional rhytidectomy.[40] Data from 10 patients showed that waterjet parotidectomy using a nozzle size of 120 microns and jet pressures from 30 to 50 bar did not cause any facial nerve dysfunction.[36] Data obtained from a pilot study comparing 30 patients undergoing waterjet tonsillectomy with a 120 microns diameter nozzle at pressures up to 60 bar with 30 patients treated by conventional tonsillectomy showed a significant reduction of intraoperative and postoperative bleeding in the waterjet group.[40] At the authors' institution, waterjet is routinely used for debridement of severe maxillofacial wounds and necrotic infections. Newer hybrid systems combining waterjet dissection and coagulation into a single device may prove valuable and efficient for the excision of salivary gland tumors.

The potential role of waterjet cutting for neck dissection for malignant disease remains obscure, as there is little data on the effect of waterjet on lymph nodes. In one report of patients undergoing retroperitoneal lymph node dissection for testicular cancer, it was shown that at pressures of 20 bar, the lymph node capsules remain intact.[41] The optimal range for fatty tissue dissection has been described to lie between 30 and 40 bar.[42] Studies aimed specifically at lymph node integrity in response to pressures required to cut through

fat, glandular parenchyma, and nerves of the head and neck are needed before using waterjet for neck dissection and lymphadenectomy for malignancies.

RAPID EVAPORATIVE IONIZATION MASS SPECTROMETRY: THE INTELLIGENT SURGICAL KNIFE
Technology

REIMS allows for real-time analysis of tissues and detection of malignancy while the tissue is being cut. This advantage of real-time intraoperative analysis, coupled with no requirement for sample preparation, gives the technology significant potential and clinical utility. The ability to distinguish between normal tissue and tumor is accomplished by chemical or metabolomic analysis of the surgical plume generated by diathermy or lasers. Heat causes sublimation of tissues from solid into a gas phase and the surgical smoke becomes a source of aerosolized lipids. A spectral profile of the lipids is created by REIMS, which incorporates a multivariate statistical analytical software. The software pulls from an online library of tissue-specific spectral profiles or "fingerprints" and algorithms allow for the characterization of the spectral profile into tissue diagnostic data.[43]

The average time from activation of the electro-surgical knife to completion of the analysis and phenotyping of the tissues as "normal" or "tumor" was shown to be as low as 1.80 seconds intraoperatively.[43] More recent iterations reduced this analysis time down to 0.7 seconds (Dhanda J. 2019; Personal communication. Ongoing studies at Queen Victoria Hospital, East Grinstead, United Kingdom.). The intelligent knife or "iknife" technology incorporates a conventional diathermy tip, a plume-collecting mechanism, and an attached mass spectrometer with a computer as a single setup (**Fig. 6**A). This technology and setup are under investigation to combine it with robotic and transoral laser techniques in head and neck cancer in the United Kingdom (Dhanda J. 2019; Personal communication. Ongoing studies at Queen Victoria Hospital, East Grinstead, United Kingdom.). The greatest benefit this real-time analysis can offer is in the detection of tumor cells at margins of resection during surgery. This technology could have the potential to reduce recurrence

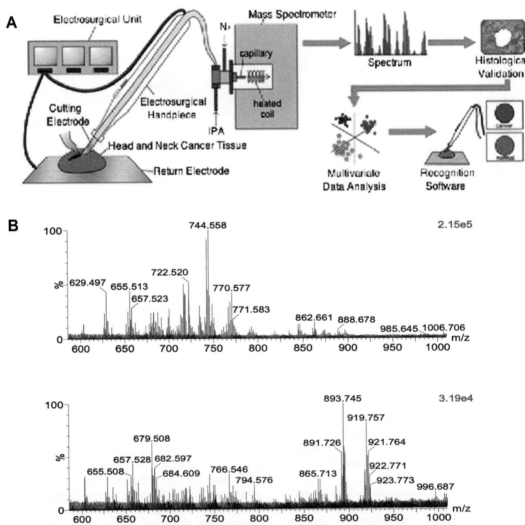

Fig. 6. (*A*) Setup and workflow diagram showing experimental iknife technology. (*B*) REIMS spectra showing different patterns and peak intensities in normal tissues (*top*) and that of oral squamous cell carcinoma (*bottom*). Such differences correspond to the different lipodomes of normal versus cancerous tissue. ([A] *Adapted from* St John, ER, Balog J, McKenzie JS, et al. Rapid evaporative ionisation mass spectrometry of electrosurgical vapours for the identification of breast pathology: towards an intelligent knife for breast cancer surgery. Breast Cancer Res. 2017;19(1)59; with permission. The original article is an open access article distributed under the terms of the Creative Commons Attribution License (http://creativecommons.org/licenses/by/2.0), which permits unrestricted use, distribution, and reproduction in any medium, provided the original work is properly cited; and [B] *Courtesy of* Jagtar Dhanda, Queen Victoria Hospital, East Grinstead, United Kingdom.)

due to positive surgical margins as well as to reduce operative time by potentially eliminating time spent for the assessment of frozen sections.

The ability of REIMS technology to differentiate between cancerous and normal adjacent tissues has been shown in lesions of the breast,[43] ovaries (Dhanda J. 2019; Personal communication. Ongoing studies at Queen Victoria Hospital, East Grinstead, United Kingdom.), colon,[44] brain,[45] and oral cavity lesions.[46] The intelligent knife was able to differentiate between colorectal carcinoma and adjacent normal tissue with an overall accuracy of 94.4% in patients undergoing endoscopy using a modified endoscopic REIMS snare.[45] In ovarian cancer, the intelligent knife was able to differentiate between cancer and normal ovary with 97.4% sensitivity and 100% specificity.[44] In patients with breast cancer, normal breast tissue was differentiated from tumor with 93.4% sensitivity and 94.9% specificity.[43] In neurosurgery, the intelligent knife was able to distinguish between World Health Organization Grade II and Grade IV tumors intraoperatively, thus showing the potential of its application in brain tumors as well.[47]

The underlying concept is that cancerous cells, as well as different types of cancers of the same tissue type, are composed of different compositions and ratios of lipids compared with normal tissues, each producing unique spectral profiles. In ovarian cancer, for example, spectra of cancerous tissues show a higher concentration of phosphatidylethanolamine compared with borderline and normal tissues.[44] With regard to colon pathology, normal mucosa expresses a relatively high ratio of plasmalogens and triacylglycerols, adenomas express ceramides, and carcinoma expresses long-chain phosphatidylserines.[45] Similar differences in lipid composition have been shown in breast and brain tumors compared with adjacent normal tissues.[43,47] The intelligent knife can therefore function as an intraoperative margin assessment tool or as a diagnostic molecular sampling tool for the identification of various tumors. Because it has been shown that there is high sensitivity and specificity when comparing spectral data from fresh with those from defrosted samples,[43] it will be possible to construct spectral profiles of different tumors of multiple tissue types and organs using archived frozen samples.

Applications in Oral and Maxillofacial Surgery

This technology has great potential in head and neck surgery beyond just margin control during ablative procedures. It could have a role in mucosal excision for unknown primary, in organ preservation techniques in laryngeal resection, as well as a role in the management of recurrence. The applications of this technology in the diagnosis of human papillomavirus and the management of dysplasia are also potential avenues for investigation.

There is little data regarding the use of the intelligent knife technology for head and neck tumors and therefore, a limited spectral library of such tumors. In a recent initial cohort study of 30 archived snap-frozen samples, iknife technology using diathermy and laser cutting was applied to obtain spectral profiles of oral cavity tumors (squamous cell carcinoma) and paired normal tissues followed by histopathologic validation of a tissue diagnosis (**Fig. 6**).[46]

Using leave-one-patient-out cross-validation showed better discrimination between snap-frozen paired tumor and normal tissue using laser (95% specificity and 98% sensitivity) compared with diathermy (95% specificity and 92% sensitivity).[46] The only misclassified sample in the laser group had a few strands of cytologically malignant cells in the final histopathologic validation. An ongoing follow-up study of 80 tumors paired with normal tissue, fat, and muscle analysis using both laser and diathermy showed an overall diagnostic accuracy of 96% (Dhanda J. 2019; Personal communication. Ongoing studies at Queen Victoria Hospital, East Grinstead, United Kingdom.). This work is now being developed to combine iknife technology with robotic surgery in a pilot study for a clinical trial (Dhanda J. 2019; Personal communication. Ongoing studies at Queen Victoria Hospital, East Grinstead, United Kingdom.). Future work is needed for the development of libraries of REIMS spectral profiles of multiple head and neck tumors.

REFERENCES

1. Lucibelle M. This month in physics history 2019. Available at: https://www.aps.org/publications/apsnews/201403/physicshistory.cfm. Accessed July 2, 2019.
2. Genovese M. Ultrasound transducers. J Diagn Med Sonogr 2016;32:48–53.
3. Feil W. Technology and clinical application of ultrasonic dissection. Minim Invasive Ther Allied Technol 2017;11:215–23.
4. Stübinger S, Stricker A, Berg B-I. Piezosurgery in implant dentistry. Clin Cosmet Investig Dent 2015;7:115–24.
5. Heinemann F, Hasan I, Kunert-Keil C, et al. Experimental and histological investigations of the bone using two different Oscillating Osteotomy techniques compared with conventional rotary osteotomy. Ann Anat 2012;194:165–70.

6. Stübinger S, Landes C, Seitz O, et al. Ultrasonic bone cutting in oral surgery: a review of 60 cases. Ultraschall Med 2008;29:66–71 [in German].

7. Rashad A, Sadr-Eshkevari P, Heiland M, et al. Intra-osseous heat generation during sonic, ultrasonic and conventional osteotomy. J Craniomaxillofac Surg 2015;43:1072–7.

8. Preti G, Martinasso G, Peirone B, et al. Cytokines and growth factors involved in the osseointegration of oral titanium implants positioned using piezo-electric bone surgery versus a drill technique: a pilot study in minipigs. J Periodontol 2007;78:716–22.

9. Al-Dajani M. Recent trends in sinus lift surgery and their clinical implications. Clin Implant Dent Relat Res 2016;18:204–12.

10. Jordi C, Mukaddam K, Lambrecht J, et al. Membrane perforation rate in lateral maxillary sinus floor augmentation using conventional rotating instruments and piezoelectric device—a meta-analysis. Int J Implant Dent 2018;4:3.

11. Vercellotti T, Paoli DS, Nevins M. The piezoelectric bony window osteotomy and sinus membrane elevation: introduction of a new technique for simplification of the sinus augmentation procedure. Int J Periodontics Restorative Dent 2001;21:561–7.

12. Crosetti E, Battiston B, Succo G. Piezosurgery in head and neck oncological and reconstructive surgery: personal experience on 127 cases. Acta Otorhinolaryngol Ital 2009;29:1–9.

13. Spinelli G, Mannelli G, Zhang Y, et al. Complex craniofacial advancement in paediatric patients: piezoelectric and traditional technique evaluation. J Craniomaxillofac Surg 2015;43:1422–7.

14. Martini M, Röhrig A, Reich R, et al. Comparison between piezosurgery and conventional osteotomy in cranioplasty with fronto-orbital advancement. J Craniomaxillofac Surg 2017;45:395–400.

15. Rossi D, Romano M, Karanxha L, et al. Bimaxillary orthognathic surgery with a conventional saw compared with the piezoelectric technique: a longitudinal clinical study. Br J Oral Maxillofac Surg 2018;56:698–704.

16. Labanca M, Azzola F, Vinci R, et al. Piezoelectric surgery: twenty years of use. Br J Oral Maxillofac Surg 2008;46:265–9.

17. Pagotto L, de Santos T, de de Vasconcellos S, et al. Piezoelectric versus conventional techniques for orthognathic surgery: systematic review and meta-analysis. J Craniomaxillofac Surg 2017;45:1607–13.

18. Silva R, Gupta R, Tartaglia G, et al. Benefits of using the ultrasonic BoneScalpelTM in temporomandibular joint reconstruction. J Craniomaxillofac Surg 2017;45:401–7.

19. Phillips CK, Hruby GW, Durak E, et al. Tissue response to surgical energy devices. Urology 2008;71:744–8.

20. Chen C, Kallakuri S, Vedpathak A, et al. The effects of ultrasonic and electrosurgery devices on nerve physiology. Br J Neurosurg 2012;26:856–63.

21. Upadhyaya A, Hu T, Meng Z, et al. Harmonic versus LigaSure hemostasis technique in thyroid surgery: a meta-analysis. Biomed Rep 2016;5:221–7.

22. Fridman G, Friedman G, Gutsol A, et al. Applied plasma medicine. Plasma Process Polym 2008;5(6):503–33.

23. Link WJ, Incropera FP, Glover JL. The plasma scalpel. Med Prog Technol 1976;4(3):123–31.

24. Glover JL, Bendick PJ, Link WJ, et al. The plasma scalpel: a new thermal knife. Lasers Surg Med 1982;2(1):101–6.

25. Available at: https://clinicaltrials.gov/ct2/show/NCT03286283. Accessed July 2, 2019.

26. Pedroso JD, Gutierrez MM, Volker KW, et al. Thermal effect of j-plasma energy in a porcine tissue model: implications for minimally invasive surgery. Surg Technol Int 2017;30:19–24.

27. Keidar M, Walk R, Shashurin A, et al. Cold plasma selectivity and the possibility of a paradigm shift in cancer therapy. Br J Cancer 2011;105(9):1295.

28. Bahls T, Frohlich FA, Hellings A, et al. Extending the capability of using waterjet in surgical interventions by the use of robotics. IEEE Trans Biomed Eng 2017;64(2):284–94.

29. Rau HG, Duessel AP, Wurzbacher S. The use of water-jet dissection in open and laparoscopic liver dissection. HPB (Oxford) 2008;10(4):275–80.

30. Keiner D, Gaab MR, Backhaus A, et al. Waterjet dissection in neurosurgery: an update after 208 procedures with special reference to surgical technique and complications. Oper Neurosurg (Hagerstown) 2010;67(2-suppl):342–54.

31. Gilling P, Anderson P, Tan A. Aquablation of the prostate for symptomatic benign prostatic hyperplasia: 1-year results. J Urol 2017;197(6):1565–72.

32. Bach T, Giannakis I, Bachmann A, et al. Aquablation of the prostate: single center results of a non-selected, consecutive patient cohort. World J Urol 2018. https://doi.org/10.1007/s00345-018-2509-y.

33. Gilling P, Reuther R, Kahokehr A, et al. Aquablation – image-guided robot-assisted waterjet ablation of the prostate: initial clinical experience. BJU Int 2016;17(6):923–9.

34. Reber M, Nussbaumer P. Effective debridement with micro water jet technology (MWT): a retrospective clinical application observation of 90 patients with acute and chronic wounds. Wound Medicine 2018;20:35–42.

35. Magritz R, Jurk V, Reusche E, et al. Water-jet dissection in parotid surgery: an experimental study in dogs. Laryngoscope 2001;111(9):1579–84.

36. Seigert R, Magritz R, Jurk V. Water-jet dissection in parotid surgery-initial clinical results. Laryngorhinootologie 2001;79(12):780–4.

37. Huang R, Yan H, Ren G, et al. Comparison of the o-type hybridknife to conventional knife in endoscopic submucosal dissection for gastric mucosal lesions. Medicine 2016;95(13):e3148.

38. Pech O. Hybrid argon plasma coagulation in patients with barrett esophagus. Gastroenterol Hepatol 2017;13(10):610–2.

39. Lorenz K, Kresz A, Maier H. Hydrodissection for tonsillectomy. Results of a pilot study-intraoperative blood loss, postoperative pain symptoms and risk of secondary hemorrhage. HNO 2005;53(5):423–7.

40. Kaye KO, Kasner S, Paprottka FJ, et al. The liquid facelift: first hands-on experience with facial water jet-assisted liposuction as an additive technique for rhytidectomy: a case series of 25 patients. J Plast Reconstr Aesthet Surg 2018;71(2):171–7.

41. Corvin S, Sturm W, Schlatter E, et al. Laparoscopic retroperitoneal lymph-node dissection with waterjet is technically feasible and safe in testis-cancer patient. J Endourol 2005;19(7):823–6.

42. Wanner M, Jakob S, Schwarzl F, et al. Water jet dissection in fatty tissue. Swiss Surg 2013;7(4):173–9.

43. St. John ER, Balog J, McKenzie JS, et al. Rapid evaporative ionisation mass spectrometry of electrochemical vapours for identification of breast pathology: towards an intelligent knife for breast cancer surgery. Breast Cancer Res 2017;19(1):59.

44. Phelps DL, Balog J, Gildea LF, et al. The surgical intelligent knife distinguishes normal, borderline, and malignant gynaecological tissues using rapid evaporative ionization mass spectrometry (REIMS). Br J Cancer 2018;118(10):1349–58.

45. Alexander J, Gildea L, Balog J, et al. A novel methodology for in vivo endoscopic phenotyping of colorectal cancer based on real-time analysis if the mucosal lipodome: a prospective observational study of the iknife. Surg Endosc 2017;31(3):1361–70.

46. Dhanda J, Schache A, Robinson M, et al. iKnife rapid evaporative ionisation mass spectrometry (REIMS) technology in head and neck surgery. A ex vivo feasibility study. Br J Oral Maxillofac Surg 2017;55(10):e61.

47. Vaqas B, Balog J, Roncaroli F, et al. iKnife in neurosurgery: intraoperative real-time, in vivo biochemical characterization of brain tumors with high spatial resolution. Cancer Res 2015;75(15-suppl):LB-287.

Minimally Invasive Endoscopic Oral and Maxillofacial Surgery

Mohamed A. Hakim, DDS[a], Joseph P. McCain, DMD[a], David Y. Ahn, DMD[b], Maria J. Troulis, DDS, MSc[a],*

KEYWORDS

- Arthroscopy • Endoscopy • Minimally invasive • Sialoendoscopy

KEY POINTS

- Technological advances have allowed for specialized endoscopes and instruments for use in the maxillofacial region.
- Advanced surgical arthroscopy of the temporomandibular joint can predictably replace traditional open approaches.
- Endoscopy can be used to approach the ramus condyle unit and the orbit.
- Sialoendoscopy can significantly reduce the need for salivary gland excision for obstructive salivary gland disease.

INTRODUCTION TO THE TECHNOLOGY

Minimally invasive surgery (MIS) can be referred to as *endoscopic surgery*, *less invasive surgery*, *video-assisted surgery*, *telescopic surgery*, and *minimal-access surgery*. It can also be broadly defined as *the discipline of surgical innovation combined with modern technology*. As Hunter and Sackier,[1] fathers of laparoscopic surgery, stated: "[t]he role of technology in minimally invasive surgery has been to miniaturize our eyes and extend our hands to perform microscopic and macroscopic operations in places that could previously be reached only with large incisions."

Using endoscopy allows for direct visualization through natural orifices or smaller incisions that are distant to the surgical site. Advances in technology allow for the development of smaller endoscopes and endoscopic instruments for operations in the maxillofacial region. Regardless of the name, MIS has been well accepted (and requested) by patients because of the decreased morbidity, shorter hospital stay, and quicker return to normal function, as compared with standard, maximally invasive techniques.[2]

Endoscopy was first introduced in 1806 by Philipp Bozzini, who created the first internally lit device to inspect the interior of the human body. His instrument, the "Lichtleiter" (*light conductor*), used a candle with angled mirrors for illumination.[3] French urologist, Antonin Jean Desormeaux, in 1853 performed an endoscopic operation with what he termed the "endoscope."[4] The first publication on arthroscopy (then called "arthro-endoscopy") came from Dr Eugen Bircher,[5] who used a laparoscope in a knee joint using nitrogen gas to distend the optical cavity. Oral and maxillofacial surgeon, Masatoshi Onishi, was first to perform temporomandibular joint (TMJ) arthroscopy using an arthroscope developed by Masaki Watanabe, a Japanese orthopedic surgeon. Since then, oral and maxillofacial surgeons, Onishi, Holmlund,

Disclosure Statement: This work was funded in part, by Fellowship Grants from DePuy Synthes (Raynham, MA) and KLS Martin (Jacksonville, FL), OMFS Education and Research Fund (Boston, MA), Lynn Foundation (AZ) and the WC Guralnick (Haseotes-Bentas) Fund.
[a] Department of Oral and Maxillofacial Surgery, Massachusetts General Hospital, 55 Fruit Street, Warren 1201, Boston, MA 02114, USA; [b] 3287 Congressional CT, Fairfield, CA 94534, USA
* Corresponding author.
E-mail address: mtroulis@partners.org

Murakami, McCain, and Sanders, have further popularized TMJ arthroscopy and are considered the pioneers of this field.[6]

Interest in the minimally invasive approach to the ramus condyle unit (RCU) began in the late 1990s and early 2000s with Lee, Mueller, Schmelzeisen, Kellman, and Troulis.[7,8] Natural orifice surgery was introduced in the 1990s, as Konisgsberger, Nahlieli, Katz, and Marchal applied endoscopy to enter the salivary ducts to treat salivary gland obstruction.[9]

BIOLOGIC BASIS

MIS offers faster recovery, fewer complications, and shorter hospital stay.[2] An experimental study on Yucatan minipigs compared the postoperative edema associated with transoral vertical ramus osteotomy to endoscopic-assisted vertical ramus osteotomy using a small submandibular incision and found that the endoscopic approach resulted in less postoperative edema at 24 hours postoperatively.[10] Small incisions with minimal tissue manipulation may allow for faster recovery and reduced postoperative discomfort when compared with traditional surgical techniques.

EQUIPMENT SETUP

The *endoscopy tower* includes the *camera*, the *light source*, the *video processor*, the *monitor*, the *coupler*, and the *endoscope*. The optical characteristics include the *field of view*: the angle drawn from the tip of the rigid endoscope to the extreme edge of the field. This angle is reduced by 40% when used in a fluid medium as opposed to air. The *direction of view* is the angle projected between the long axis of the rigid endoscope and the line through the center of the image being visualized. The angle of the scope usually pertains to the latter. Endoscopes used in the head and neck region are 0°, 10°, 30°, 45°, and 70°. Focal length is the distance, in focus, between the object and the distal end of the scope. The *optical cavity* is the space where the endoscope is inserted to visualize and operate. It can be a natural cavity (eg, the maxillary sinus), generated (eg, the subperiosteal space), or a combination of both (eg, insufflated joint space in arthroscopy).

Commonly used endoscopes can be categorized into flexible, rigid, and semirigid. Flexible endoscopes are used for procedures such as gastrointestinal endoscopy and laryngoscopy. Rigid endoscopes are used for procedures like arthroscopy, rhinoscopy, and sinuscopy. Semirigid endoscopes are commonly used for sialoendoscopy.

APPLICATIONS IN MAXILLOFACIAL SURGERY

MIS, in other fields, has contributed to the armamentarium of arthroscopy, endoscopy, and sialoendoscopy. Common teachings include the entry or access port, working port, optical cavity, and endoscopic landmarks.

Temporomandibular Joint Arthroscopy

Arthroscopy is used for the diagnosis and management of multiple TMJ disorders. The arthroscopes are usually rigid and small (1.2–2.4 mm). A 30° arthroscope is typically used for diagnostic or advanced surgical arthroscopy. The optical cavity is the joint space that is initially insufflated before the puncture and then maintained via irrigation.

There are different levels of arthroscopy according to the *McCain Classification*, described as:

- *Level I*: A single-puncture arthroscopy into the posterior pouch of the superior joint space along with an outflow needle. This allows for lysis and lavage or arthroscopic arthrocentesis in addition to the diagnostic value of seeing the joint anatomy (**Fig. 1**).
- *Level II*: A double-puncture arthroscopy, where the arthroscopic cannula is inserted into the posterior pouch and the operative cannula is introduced into the anterior recess of the joint using the triangulation technique.

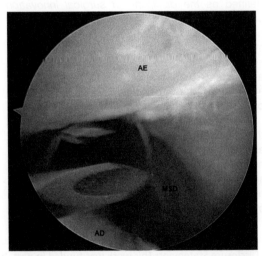

Fig. 1. Level I arthroscopy of the left TMJ. A single puncture into the posterior pouch of the joint with an outflow needle for arthroscopic arthrocentesis. The arrow typically points anteriorly for orientation. Arthroscopic view of the articular eminence (AE), the medial synovial drape (MSD), and the articular disc (AD). Notice the chondromalacia on the AE and the disc fragmentation.

This operative cannula gives the ability to perform operative procedures, such as

- o Synovial biopsy to assist in the diagnosis of the underlying pathologic condition (**Fig. 2**)
- o Lysis of adhesions under direct visualization
- o Debridement of arthritic joints aiding in creating a larger joint space and smoother surfaces to allow for improved function
- o Retrodiscal contracture to reduce redundant synovium or treat recurrent mandibular dislocation from hypermobility
- o Targeted deposition of medication through the operative cannula for disease modification
- Level III:
  - o Arthroscopic disc reduction and fixation (discopexy), which includes myotomy of the lateral pterygoid attachment to the anteriorly displaced disc, disc reduction, retrodiscal contracture, and disc fixation (**Fig. 3**)
  - o Advanced debridement of Wilkes V and fibrous ankylosis

Discussion

Traditional open operations for discopexy and recurrent mandibular dislocation are being replaced with minimally invasive arthroscopic surgeries.[11–13] Creating microfractures on articular surfaces to stimulate fibrocartilage formation is a promising area of research for treatment of chondromalacia of the TMJ.[14] There are no significant studies that directly compare advanced and single- puncture (level I) arthroscopy. Martin Granizo and colleagues[15] performed advanced arthroscopy on 659 patients. Only 5.9% of the patients required additional arthroscopic intervention, and

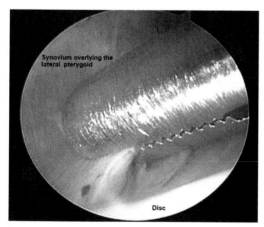

Fig. 2. Level II arthroscopy of the right TMJ. Through the operative cannula, a tissue grasper is used to obtain a sample of the medial synovium of the anterior recess of the superior joint space.

only 4 patients failed to improve from the second procedure. Two of those patients underwent open arthrotomy. Breik and colleagues[16] showed that the rate of reoperation after level I arthroscopy was 22% of 167 patients. This difference in outcome could be explained by the more definitive nature of double-puncture arthroscopy. A randomized clinical trial comparing level I to advanced arthroscopy done by the same surgeon is needed to provide definitive evidence on the matter.

Endoscopic Maxillofacial Surgery

Traditional approaches to the maxillofacial region have been maximally invasive. The introduction of endoscopy allows access to be made smaller and distant to the targeted area or through the natural orifice (eg, the mouth). Oral and maxillofacial endoscopy has been used to access the RCU, maxillary sinus, and orbital floors.

The most common approach for MIS has been the RCU. Either intraoral or remotely placed extraoral incisions reduce risk to the facial nerve injury. The rate of temporary facial nerve injury with standard open approaches has been reported to be as high as 17%,[17] whereas it can be as low as 0% and 2.5% to 6.5% with the extraoral and transoral endoscopic approaches, respectively.[8,18,19] The facial nerve weakness reported, with the latter, was that of the buccal branch, which is less detrimental than marginal mandibular and frontal branch injuries owing to cross-innervation with the zygomatic branch, which can be as high as 70%.[20] Despite being uncommon, permanent facial nerve injury has been reported with open approaches,[17] whereas it has not been noted with endoscopic procedures.

Endoscopes are usually rigid, 30°, and can range from 2.7 to 4.0 mm in diameter. The extraoral approaches require a 1.5-cm submandibular incision in a natural neck crease.[8] Intraoral approaches include an incision of approximately 1.5 cm in the mucosa over the anterior edge of the ascending ramus.[21] The optical cavity is created with subperiosteal dissection and retraction to allow for insertion of the scope and the instruments. Landmarks for endoscopy include extraoral markings on the skin and endoscopic visualization of the angle and posterior border of the mandible, ascending ramus, condylar neck, sigmoid notch, and coronoid process.

The transoral approach has applicability for the subcondylar fractures (**Fig. 4**), whereas the extraoral approach can be used for anything related to the RCU. Procedures that can be performed

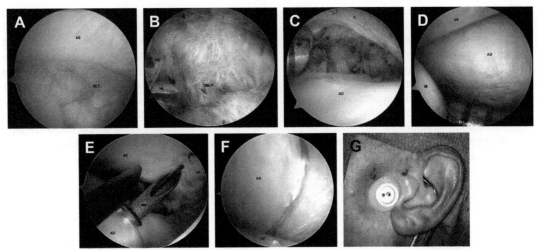

Fig. 3. Level III arthroscopic discopexy of the left TMJ; open mouth position demonstrates retrodiscal tissue (RDT) under the AE, indicating an anteriorly dislocated disc. Notice the hyperemia of the RDT (*A*). The operative cannula (OC) is inserted into the most anterolateral portion of the anterior recess, and holmium laser (HL) is used to cut the attachment of the superior belly of the lateral pterygoid (SBLP) to the AD (*B*). Zoomed out photograph demonstrates separation of the synovium (S) from the AD, which gave access to the lateral pterygoid muscle, which has been incised in this picture (*C*). The OC is used to reduce the AD so it lies under the AE. Irrigation bubbles (IB) can form during arthroscopy (*D*). The RDT has been reduced posteriorly under the glenoid fossa (GF). The disc is held in reduction with the OC, while a meniscus mender (MM) is inserted through the skin to lightly contact the condyle and then directed superiorly through the posterolateral portion of the disc; then, a 28-gauge wire is passed through it. Another MM is inserted directly into the superior joint space, and a lasso is used to capture the wire. The MMs are withdrawn to leave the 2 ends of the wire on the external surface of preauricular region (*E*). The OC is moved above the wire to hold the disc in reduction (*F*), while the wire is externally tightened through a button (*G*). The wire and button are typically left in place for 2 to 3 weeks and then removed in office.

from an extraoral approach include condylectomy and costochondral grafts, coronoidectomy, vertical ramus osteotomy/fixation, biopsy, and Open reduction internal fixation (ORIF) of subcondylar fractures.

Endoscopy can be used for transantral orbital floor reconstruction to help guide the plate placement through the traditional periorbital approaches.[22] The use of an endoscope to visualize the orbital floor plate makes it easier to find the posterior orbital ledge with less dissection of the orbital tissues, which can lead to less swelling and postoperative discomfort. It also ensures the stability of the plate and the proper positioning. A pure endoscopic transantral approach can also be used to repair orbital floor defects.[23] A 0°, 30°, 45°, or 70° endoscope is used. The maxillary sinus is a natural optical cavity (**Fig. 5**).

Sialoendoscopy

The traditional management of obstructive salivary gland disease had been excision of the submandibular or parotid glands. Such approach comes with the morbidity of facial incisions, the scarring and the risk of complications like Frey syndrome, sialocele, great auricular nerve numbness, salivary fistula, or injury of the hypoglossal, lingual, and facial nerves.[24,25] Sialoendoscopy has become a minimally invasive alternative.[9] Sialoendoscopy is indicated for diagnostic and operative management of obstructive salivary gland disease (eg, stones, including those proximally located near the hilum, strictures, and kinks). Only 20% of obstructive sialadenitis are due to stones,[26] whereas other causes can be strictures, kinks, polyps, foreign bodies, or mucus plugs.[27]

The endoscopes used for sialoendoscopy are usually semirigid with a 0° to 10° angle. The size of the scope can range from 0.9 to 1.6 mm. Larger endoscopes can allow for operative sialoendoscopy and instrumentation with baskets that are used to remove stones, graspers that can remove debris, and lasers than can break down larger stones. The natural orifice of the duct is used for the access. The optical cavity is the duct itself, which is insufflated via irrigation.

The procedure can be done under local or general anesthesia, starting with examination to inspect for stones, salivary flow, or purulent

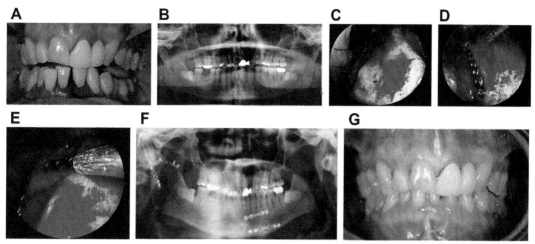

Fig. 4. Transoral endoscopically assisted repair of a right subcondylar fracture. A 50-year-old man sustained a left mandibular body and a right subcondylar fracture during a baseball game. Malocclusion photograph (*A*). Panoramic radiograph demonstrated the right subcondylar and the left body fractures (*B*). After maxillomandibular fixation and fixation of the left body with two 2.0 plates, a sagittal split osteotomy incision was made on the right side and a 4-mm 30° endoscope was inserted to visualize the mandibular ramus (MR), coronoid process (CP), condylar neck (CN); then the fracture was reduced (*C*). A 2.0 plate was used to fixate the fracture along the posterior border (*D*). Then a midface plate was used under the sigmoid notch for additional stability (*E*). Postoperative radiograph showed adequate restoration of the RCU height (*F*). Three months follow-up demonstrated a stable postoperative occlusion (*G*).

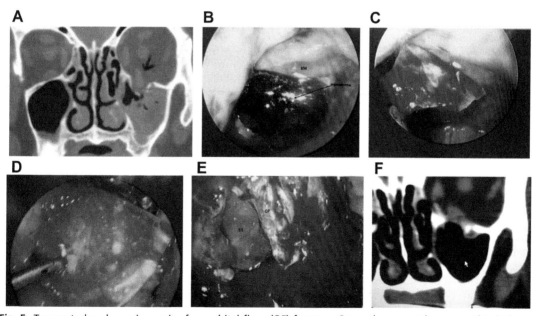

Fig. 5. Transantral endoscopic repair of an orbital floor (OF) fracture. Coronal computed tomographic (CT) scan showed a left OF fracture with herniation of the orbital contents (arrow head) (*A*). A modified Caldwell Luc incision was made followed by an antrostomy large enough to allow for insertion of the implant. Endoscopic view showed healthy sinus mucosa (SM) adjacent to a hematoma with positive pulse test indicating herniation of the orbital contents (*B*). The sinus roof was demucosalized, and loose fragments of bone were removed (*C*). The orbital contents were preserved and reduced superiorly; then a silastic sheet (SS) was inserted to reconstruct the OF (*D*). Once inserted through the OF, the SS unfolded to achieve stable reconstruction of the defect (*E*). Postoperative CT scan showed adequate reduction of the orbital contents (*F*).

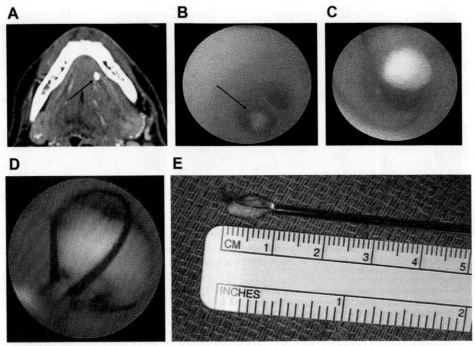

Fig. 6. Operative sialoendoscopy of the left submandibular gland. An axial CT scan of the neck showed an approximately 6 × 5-mm stone in the left submandibular duct (arrow head) (*A*). The duct orifice was dilated until a 1.6-mm 10° sialoscope was inserted, and the stone was visualized proximally at the hilum (arrow head) (*B*). Then, a basket was passed through the operative channel of the sialoscope proximal to the stone and opened (*C*). An example of how the basket is gently closed to capture the stone without fragmentation (*D*). Then, the sialoscope and the basket were simultaneously withdrawn. Ex vivo view of a stone attached to the basket and the sialoscope (*E*).

discharge. Afterward, sequential dilation of the duct is performed depending on the size of the endoscope being used. The endoscope is inserted and advanced proximally. Once a stone is localized and removed, the ductal system is reexamined for secondary stones (**Fig. 6**). The ductal system, in the absence of a sialolith, is examined for kinks, strictures, or other causes of obstruction as far proximally past the hilum as possible.

WORKFLOW

When clinical scenarios present themselves in a minimally invasive maxillofacial surgery practice, the diagnosis is made, and the treatment needed is decided. Then a decision is made whether the treatment can be done endoscopically. With TMJs, it is usually beneficial to give the patient the benefit of a minimally invasive attempt before considering open arthrotomy. When it comes to the RCU, the experience of the surgical team determines their ability to take on more difficult procedures endoscopically. For example, a medially displaced subcondylar fracture would be attempted endoscopically by

experienced endoscopists before converting to open, whereas a low fracture would be ideal for a beginner.

Role assignment in endoscopy is critical to the workflow. With advanced arthroscopy, the primary surgeon needs 2 surgical assistants. Although 1 assistant distracts the mandible and assists with instrument exchange, the other assists with irrigation. With subcondylar fractures, the endoscopist's main role is to enhance the optical cavity, expose the fracture, and assist with the reduction; meanwhile, the first assistant is responsible for the fixation. With sialoendoscopy, the assistant is needed to pass the operative instruments through the endoscopic channel to remove stones and debris.

SUMMARY

As the modern world becomes driven by technology, surgeons should expand their interest and keep abreast of such advances to further develop the specialty. Future innovations and additional research have the potential to further expand clinical application of minimally invasive techniques in oral and maxillofacial surgery.

REFERENCES

1. Hunter JG, Sackier JM. Minimally invasive high tech surgery; into the 21st century. In: Hunter JG, Sackier JM, editors. Minimally invasive surgery. New York: McGraw-Hill; 1993. p. 3–6.
2. Li H, Wang GS. Laparoscopic VS open hepatectomy for hepatolithiasis: an updated systematic review and meta-analysis. World J Gastroenterol 2017; 23(43):7791–806.
3. Verger-Kuhnke AB, Reuter MA, Beccaria ML. La biografía de Philipp Bozzini (1773-1809) un idealista de la endoscopia.
4. Paraskeva PA, Nduka CC, Darzi A. The evolution of laparoscopic surgery. Minimally Invasive Therapy 1994;3(2):69–75.
5. Bircher E. Die arthroendoskopie. Zentralbl Chir 1921;48:1460–1.
6. Nitzan DW, Dolwick MF, Heft MW. Arthroscopic lavage and lysis of the temporomandibular joint: a change in perspective. J Oral Maxillofac Surg 1990;49:799–901.
7. Kellman RM. Endoscopically assisted repair of subcondylar fractures of the mandible an evolving technique. Arch Facial Plast Surg 2003;5:244–50.
8. Troulis MJ, Kaban LB. Endoscopic approach to the ramus/condyle unit: clinical applications. J Oral Maxillofac Surg 2001;59(5):503–9.
9. Papadaki ME, McCain JP, Kim K, et al. Interventional sialoendoscopy: early clinical results. J Oral Maxillofac Surg 2008;66:954–62.
10. Williams WB, Troulis MJ, Kaban LB. A comparison of postoperative edema after intraoral vs endoscopic mandibular ramus osteotomy. J Oral Maxillofac Surg 2003;61(8S). 61a-2.
11. Liu X, Zheng J, Cai X, et al. Techniques of Yang's arthroscopic discopexy for temporomandibular joint rotational anterior disc displacement. Int J Oral Maxillofac Surg 2019;48(6):769–78.
12. Ohnishi M. Arthroscopic surgery for hypermobility and recurrent mandibular dislocation. Oral Maxillofac Surg Clin North Am 1989;1:153–64.
13. Torres DE, McCain JP. Arthroscopic electrothermal capsulorrhaphy for the treatment of recurrent temporomandibular joint dislocation. Int J Oral Maxillofac Surg 2012;41:681–9.
14. Knutsen G, Drogset JO, Engebretsen L, et al. A randomized trial comparing autologous chondrocyte implantation with microfracture. Findings at five years. J Bone Joint Surg Am 2007;89:2105–12.
15. Martin GR, Correa Muñoz DC, Varela Reyes E. Rearthroscopy of the temporomandibular joint: a retrospective study of 600 arthroscopies. J Craniomaxillofac Surg 2018;46(9):1555–60.
16. Breik O, Devrukhkar V, Dimitroulis G. Temporomandibular joint (TMJ) arthroscopic lysis and lavage: outcomes and rate of progression to open surgery. J Craniomaxillofac Surg 2016;44:1988–95.
17. Ellis E, McFadden D, Simon P, et al. Surgical complications with open treatment of mandibular condylar process fractures. J Oral Maxillofac Surg 2000;58: 950–8.
18. Aneshur V, Kulkarni K, Shetty S, et al. Clinical outcomes of endoscopic vs. retromandibular approach for the treatment of condylar fractures–a randomized clinical trial. Oral Surg Oral Med Oral Pathol Oral Radiol 2018. https://doi.org/10.1016/j.oooo. 2018.12.007.
19. Blumer M, Guggenbühl T, Wagner MEH, et al. Outcomes of surgically treated fractures of the condylar process by an endoscopic assisted transoral approach. J Oral Maxillofac Surg 2019;77:133.e1-9.
20. Gosain AK. Surgical anatomy of the facial nerve. Clin Plast Surg 1995;22:241.
21. Akdag O, Yildiran G, Abaci M, et al. Endoscopic-assisted treatment combined with transoral and transbuccal approach to mandibular subcondylar fractures. J Oral Maxillofac Surg 2018;76:831.e1-5.
22. Moura LB, Filho VA. Reconstruction of orbital floor defects assisted by transantral endoscopy. Oral Maxillofac Surg 2017;21(1):65–8.
23. Miloro M. Endoscopically assisted repair of orbital floor fractures. Arch Facial Plast Surg 2002;4(2): 124–5.
24. Infante-Cossio P, Gonzalez-Cardero E, Garcia-Perla-Garcia A, et al. Complications after superficial parotidectomy for pleomorphic adenoma. Med Oral Patol Oral Cir Bucal 2018;23(4):e485–92.
25. Milton CM, Thomas BM, Bickerton RC. Morbidity study of submandibular gland excision. Ann R Coll Surg Engl 1986;68(3):148–50.
26. Koch M, Zenk J, Bozzato A, et al. Sialoscopy in cases of unclear swelling of major salivary glands. Otolaryngol Head Neck Surg 2005;133(6):863–8.
27. Strychowsky JE, Sommer DD, Gupta MK, et al. Sialendoscopy for the management of obstructive salivary gland disease, a systematic review and meta-analysis. Arch Otolaryngol Head Neck Surg 2012; 138(NO. 6).

Adjunctive Strategies for Benign Maxillofacial Pathology

Zachary S. Peacock, DMD, MD

KEYWORDS

- Odontogenic keratocyst • Giant cell lesion • Ameloblastoma • Benign jaw tumor
- Keratocystic odontogenic tumor • Giant cell granuloma • Unicystic ameloblastoma

KEY POINTS

- Benign aggressive lesions of the maxillofacial region, such as the odontogenic keratocyst, giant cell lesion, and ameloblastoma, often require surgical treatment similar to treatment of malignancies.
- Strategies exist for less invasive or adjunctive treatment, with varying results.
- The identification of the genetic profile of these cysts and neoplasms may make medical treatment of traditionally surgical disease possible.

INTRODUCTION

Benign cysts and neoplasms of the maxillofacial skeleton can be locally aggressive, resulting in destruction of surrounding structures. Lesions such as the odontogenic keratocyst (OKC) and ameloblastoma have considerable rates of recurrence and may require morbid treatment to prevent recurrence. As the pathogenesis of benign lesions has become better understood, less invasive and more directed treatment strategies have been used with evolving success.

Advances in less invasive and adjunctive treatment of benign maxillofacial cysts and neoplasms are reviewed here with an update on future management strategies for 3 common lesions encountered by oral and maxillofacial surgeons.

ODONTOGENIC KERATOCYST

The OKC is familiar to oral and maxillofacial surgeons is the prototype lesion for attempts at reducing surgical morbidity. While resection with negative margins can eliminate or minimize recurrence, the benign histology of the OKC has prompted attempts at less morbid treatment.[1–7] Enucleation as sole treatment of an OKC is associated with high recurrence rates.[8–10] The lesion often presents as multilocular with a thin, friable lining, and a tendency to be associated with tooth roots which makes access difficult and often results in incomplete removal.[11] The lesion has a tendency to form 'daughter cysts' beyond the main osseous cavity not visible after enucleation. Any remaining cells and even the overlying mucosa can result in a recurrence in the short or long term.[12]

Advances in adjunctive treatment that can be used in addition to enucleation have helped reduce recurrence of OKC. Adjunctive treatment is highly variable among practitioners and outcomes vary widely in the literature. Goals of treatment are to eliminate the residual cells not seen after enucleation (eg, around tooth roots and within daughter cysts). Options for adjunctive treatment include, but are not limited to, physical destruction via peripheral ostectomy, cryotherapy, or chemical treatment with

Disclosure: The author has nothing to disclose.
Department of Oral and Maxillofacial Surgery, Massachusetts General Hospital, Harvard School of Dental Medicine, 55 Fruit Street Warren 1201, Boston, MA 02421, USA
E-mail address: zpeacock@partners.org

Oral Maxillofacial Surg Clin N Am 31 (2019) 569–578
https://doi.org/10.1016/j.coms.2019.07.002

fixative agents (ie, Carnoy solution).[13] A technique used for large lesions is decompression by maintaining an opening from the lesion to the oral cavity. This technique is performed via marsupialization or stenting with a conduit/drain.[14–16] The resultant smaller lesion can then be subjected to enucleation/adjunctive treatment.[15]

Peripheral Ostectomy

Once a lesion is enucleated and visibly absent, additional mechanical bone removal can be used to extend the osseous cavity and reduce recurrence.[16] Theoretically, removing an additional 1 to 2 mm of bone peripherally with a carbide bur can eliminate cells or daughter cysts beyond the osseous cavity. Consistent and complete removal can be aided by application of methylene blue to the cavity with bone removal until the dye is gone.[17] Application of this technique around tooth roots and the inferior alveolar nerve is challenging and may be the reason for recurrences.

Cryotherapy

Application of liquid nitrogen to osseous cavities after enucleation has been shown to reduce recurrence rates and reduce the need for resection.[18,19] Freezing the residual bony cavity in this way results in cell death to a depth of up to 1.5 mm.[20] The surrounding soft tissue and other structures must be carefully protected to avoid inadvertent freezing and tissue necrosis. Access to all areas of a bony cavity can be challenging when dispensed via a metal cannula. An advantage of this technique is the ability to treat tooth roots and bone around the inferior alveolar nerve, where use of a surgical drill can be limited. Although paresthesia results, reasonable recovery can be expected.[21] Depending on the size of the lesion, with circumferential necrosis, the mandible can be weakened and at risk for fracture.[22] For this reason, it may be necessary to perform autogenous bone grafting, limit the patient's diet, or apply maxillomandibular fixation.

Chemical Treatment

Chemical treatment of the bony cavity has been effective in reducing recurrence rates compared with enucleation alone.[23,24] The most commonly reported agent, Carnoy solution (absolute alcohol, chloroform, ferric chloride, glacial acetic acid) is controversial because chloroform was classified as a carcinogen and its use in compounded therapeutic agents was banned by the US Food and Drug Administration in 1992.[25] Reports on 'modified Carnoy' solution, not containing chloroform, seem to confirm that chloroform is necessary for its success.[26] Despite its success, it seems that alternatives to chemical fixation should be used as adjunctive treatment of lesions such as the OKC.

Decompression and Stenting of Larger Lesions

Treatment of larger cystic lesions (3 cm) with enucleation/curettage and adjunctive treatment remains difficult. Access to all parts of the lesion can be challenging and typically the surrounding bone is thin or perforated, limiting ostectomy or cryotherapy. Cystic lesions increase in size because of a fluid shift toward the lumen caused by increasing osmotic gradient from cellular debris or keratin.[27,28] Maintaining an opening into the lesion then decompresses a cystic lesion, reversing this gradient and causing a resultant gradual decrease in size. This outcome can be achieved by marsupialization (ie, sewing the lining of the lesion to the oral mucosa) or using a conduit from the oral cavity into the lesion. For the OKC, the thin, friable lining makes marsupialization difficult, with the natural tendency for the wound to shrink concentrically and close. Use of a drain such as a nasal trumpet, or pediatric endotracheal tube, can be more reliable to maintain communication with the lesion.

Enthusiasm for decompression/stenting peaked with reports of its use of definitive treatment (ie, until the lesion is not seen radiographically).[29] Subsequently, recurrence rates were shown to become problematic, and enucleation and adjunctive treatment of the smaller residual lesion is now recommended.[17] Beyond the physical decrease in size of the decompressed lesion, the lining of the OKC changes after long-term decompression. The typical thin, friable membrane thickens from inflammation and has an appearance like oral mucosa.[29–32] It is then more amenable to enucleation at time of residual cystectomy (**Fig. 1**). Metaplasia may also occur with loss of cytokeratin-10 immunohistochemical expression in up to 64% of OKCs and could contribute to lower recurrence rates.[32]

Future directions

The discussed treatments for the OKC remain in everyday use, but the future likely lies with more direct treatments of this benign lesion. Ideally, medical treatment can further limit the surgical burden and allow maintenance of teeth. With the elucidation of several mutations associated with

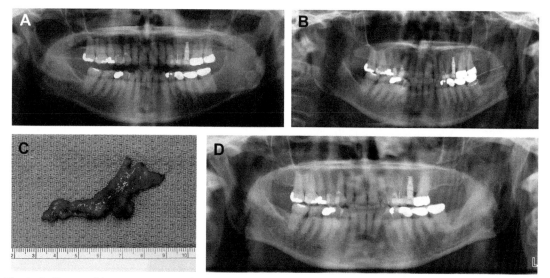

Fig. 1. A 45-year-old women presented with a large left mandibular lesion. (*A*) Intraoperative frozen section biopsy of the thin friable lesion revealed OKC, so a pediatric endotracheal tube was placed into the lesion and secure to the second molar for decompression. (*B*) Fourteen months of decompression resulted in a marked centripetal bone formation with recapitulation of the inferior alveolar nerve canal. (*C*) Residual cystectomy was then performed with cryotherapy to the osseous cavity. The lesion was thick and easy to enucleate as a single specimen. (*D*) Three-year follow-up revealed complete bone fill without evidence of recurrence.

OKCs that have existing treatment options, targeted therapy seems possible. Although the OKC has been changed from a cyst to a neoplasm and back again by the Worth Health Organization,[11,33] its mutational profile and tendency to recur are consistent with a neoplasm. Alterations in the Sonic hedgehog pathway have been reported in OKCs associated with nevoid basal cell carcinoma syndrome (NBCCS) and up to 84% of sporadic lesions.[11,34–36] The most common mutation associated with NBCCS is within the *PTCH1* gene, which produces the patched tumor suppressor protein.[34] Additional mutations have been reported in *SMO*, the gene that codes for the Smoothened protein, which activates Sonic hedgehog signaling.[36–38] It is likely that other unidentified mutations exist in this pathway in other sporadic lesions.

Existing drugs targeting the Sonic hedgehog pathway have been shown to have some effectiveness in treating advanced basal cell carcinoma[39] and those associated with NBCCS.[40] Vismodegib was shown to be effective in decreasing the size of OKCs in patients with NBCCS.[41–43] Side effects currently limit the use of a systemic chemotherapeutic agent for sporadic OKCs, but it can be expected that local or topical treatment may serve a role in lessening the surgical burden in patients with OKCs.

Ledderhof and colleagues[44] recently showed that 5-fluorouracil (5FU), an antimetabolite that may affect the sonic hedgehog pathway, may be an effective adjunct for OKCs. The investigators applied 5% 5FU to the osseous bed after enucleation with improved recurrence rate compared with modified Carnoy solution.

GIANT CELL LESIONS

The giant cell lesion (GCL) is a benign osseous neoplasm that affects the maxillofacial skeleton that remains poorly understood. Like the OKC, advances have been made in managing the GCL with methods other than the en bloc resection, which can result in significant surgical morbidity.

Various theories on the still-unknown biological origin have led to a variety of treatment options in the literature. Because giant cells are found in granulomas of foreign body reactions and sarcoidosis, GCLs have been theorized to be inflammatory in nature and steroid injections have been used in the form of intralesional injections.[45–47] Because a GCL closely resembles the brown tumor of hyperparathyroidism and can respond to calcitonin, it has been described as an endocrine lesion.[48–50] Given its dense vascularity, the GCL has also been hypothesized to be a vascular lesion and treated with interferon.[51] Although the lesion is named after the abundance of multinucleated giant cells, the neoplastic cells are most likely the mononuclear stromal cells.[52] These stromal cells recruit and activate the multinucleated giant cells, which develop the phenotype of an osteoclast.[53] Medications such as denosumab that disrupt osteoclast-mediated resorption have been used with some success.

GCLs of the maxillofacial region can be classified based on behavior.[54] Nonaggressive GCLs (<5 cm) without pain or damage to tooth roots generally respond to enucleation and curettage alone with few recurrences. Associated teeth and the inferior alveolar nerve can be spared. In contrast, aggressive GCLs recur after enucleation and curettage, which may be more difficult to perform because of their larger size.[55] The gold standard for aggressive GCLs remains resection with negative margins. Given the viable alternatives in most cases, resection is used sparingly in current practice. No consensus exists regarding other treatment options because reports in the literature often assess multiple or varying protocols and most do not describe GCLs consistently by behavior.[56]

Steroid Injections

Steroid injections have been used for GCLs given the theory that GCLs are inflammatory or reparative lesions. Primary treatment of GCLs has been reported with widely variable success rates.[45–47] Injections are difficult in multilocular or large lesions. Multiple injections are needed over weeks to months, so use in rapidly growing aggressive lesions is not possible. Intralesional steroids seem to be most effective for small, unilocular, nonaggressive lesions.

Interferon

Rapid growth and a prominent vascular component led to the theory that aggressive GCLs are the bone counterparts to the infantile hemangioma.[51,57] With this hypothesis, an antiangiogenic agent, interferon alfa-2a has been used as adjuvant treatment. In a recent study assessing its use in a tightly defined protocol over 20 years, only 6 of 45 (13.3%) patients had progression of disease or recurrence.[58] The protocol consisted of curettage of the lesion without extracting involved teeth and leaving the inferior alveolar nerve in place with subsequent subcutaneous interferon alfa-2a (3 million units per square meter) until the bony cavity fills with bone (typically 10–12 months) (**Fig. 2**). The downsides of this treatment regimen are the associated side effects of interferon and the need for enucleation. Fever and flulike symptoms can occur 24 to 48 hours after the first dose of interferon, but only 15.5% of patients in this study required stopping therapy before bone fill.[58] The use of interferon is the only adjuvant treatment that has reported long-term outcomes with a consistent protocol. For the few patients that have intolerance to interferon or develop antithyroid antibodies, bisphosphonates have been substituted with good success.[58]

Calcitonin

Because GCLs have a close resemblance to the brown tumor of hyperparathyroidism, adjuvant calcitonin has been reported as both adjuvant and primary treatment of maxillofacial GCLs.[48–50] Subcutaneous calcitonin has been reported to be successful for both nonaggressive and aggressive GCLs.[49] The primary disadvantage seems to be the delay in treatment response to calcitonin, which can be prohibitive in rapidly growing GCLs.

Denosumab

Receptor activator of nuclear factor-kappa B ligand (RANK-L) is critical to the pathway of osteoclast-mediated bone resorption. Denosumab, an antibody to RANK-L, has been developed and used to treat diseases involving bone resorption. Denosumab has had some success in both axial-appendicular and maxillofacial GCLs without operative intervention.[57,59,60] The ideal duration of treatment remains under investigation and recurrence after stopping therapy has been reported.[61] Denosumab is not currently recommended for the skeletally immature, which represents a large portion of maxillofacial GCLs. Additional studies are needed to determine the role of denosumab in the overall management of maxillofacial GCLs and its effects on epiphyseal growth.[62] Denosumab has been shown to help prevent growth and treat pain associated with fibrous dysplasia in children.[63,64] Potential serious side effects, including osteonecrosis of the jaw, have tempered the enthusiasm of oncologists for using denosumab for jaw lesions, but its efficacy is leading to greater acceptance.[65]

Future directions

Genetic studies of GCLs have revealed similarities in gene expression between maxillofacial GCLs and those affecting the long bones and spine (typically referred to as giant cell tumors).[66] Another study using whole-genome sequencing found mutations in genes coding for histone proteins (H3F3A) within stromal cells of the long bones and spine.[67] A separate study sequenced amplified polymerase chain reaction products and did not find these mutations in GCLs of the jaws.[68] Other consistent mutations have not been reported in these lesions at either location. It is not clear what role histones play in the development of these lesions and whether they would be amenable to medical therapy.

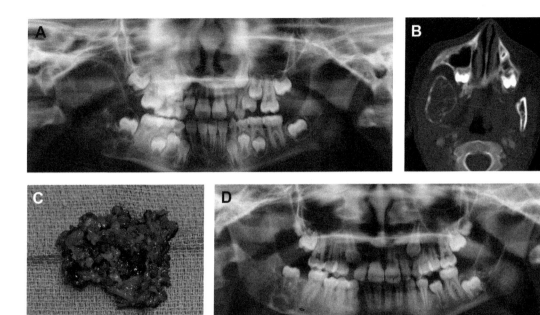

Fig. 2. An 8-year-old girl presented with a rapidly expanding painful mass of the posterior mandibular body and ramus. A panoramic radiograph (*A*) showed a multilocular radiolucent lesion involving the entire mandibular ramus unit with expansion seen on (*B*) an axial view of a computed tomography scan. (*C*) Intraoperative appearance and frozen section biopsy were consistent with a giant cell lesion so enucleation was performed, sparing the developing second molar and inferior alveolar nerve. The lesion was aggressive based on its large size, pain, and destruction of cortices, so the patient was given postoperative interferon alfa-2b for 10 months until the area had filled with bone. (*D*) A panoramic radiograph at 15 months after enucleation showed bone fill of the ramus. There was a remaining area inferior to the second molar (*arrow*) that had decreased in size and remodeled since the completion of interferon.

Although the lesions are similar histologically and radiographically, the genetic relationship between GCLs at these different locations remains unclear.[69,70] If they were found to have similar genetic aberrations, the speed at which medical therapy is developed for aggressive maxillofacial lesions would increase.

Ameloblastoma The ameloblastoma is a benign but aggressive odontogenic neoplasm that has not had significant improvements in its method of primary treatment. Although it is benign histologically, it can have rapid growth and a high rate of recurrence that requires resection with negative margins. The current standard of care is resection (segmental or marginal) with 1-cm osseous margins and 1 anatomic layer beyond the lesion (eg, periosteum). Isolated successes have been reported using less treatment, but often do not have sufficient follow-up time. Recurrence rates after resection of solid ameloblastomas have been reported between 8% and 17%.[71–73] Much higher rates (20%–90%) are seen with other less definitive treatments (eg, enucleation).[71–74]

Alternative treatments to resection are found throughout the literature.[18,75–77] Because ameloblastoma is a benign lesion, it can be difficult for surgeons and patients to accept the need for resection and the need for complex reconstruction. Unlike other benign entities, ameloblastoma is destructive and unmitigated growth, which can lead to airway compromise, rare metastases, or even death.[78–80] It has the potential to recur even decades after original treatment, which must be taken into consideration when assessing studies with limited follow-up.[81–83]

A variation of the solid ameloblastoma, the unicystic ameloblastoma, does seem to show less-aggressive behavior and less tendency to recur. Compared with the solid/multicystic ameloblastoma, the unicystic ameloblastoma may be amenable to enucleation. Robinson and Martinez[84] first reported on unicystic ameloblastoma in 1977, with a recurrence rate of 15% after enucleation, which was far less than solid/multicystic ameloblastomas. Other studies have supported the use of enucleation, with most reports having recurrence rates less than 21%.[85–87] A systematic review comparing treatments of uni-cystic ameloblastoma reported a recurrence rate of 3.6% with resection, 16% with enucleation and Carnoy solution, and 30.5% with enucleation alone.[88] Another study had 70.5% recurrence after enucleation of unicystic ameloblastoma.[89]

The relationship of the neoplastic component and the lining of a unicystic ameloblastoma has an impact on the tendency to recur and is incon-sistently reported in most studies. If the lesion is only seen in the cystic wall or projects intralumi-nally, the recurrence rate has been reported to be 10.7% with enucleation.[90] If the lesion extends beyond the cystic wall (mural involvement), the recurrence rate is much higher with enucleation and resection is recommended.

The term unicystic ameloblastoma has been inconstantly used and caution is needed before proceeding with enucleation with adjuvant treat-ment. The term may be used by radiologists based on an ameloblastoma with a single bony cavity or by pathologists if the lesion has a prominent cystic component. To confirm that an ameloblastoma is unicystic, the entire cyst wall must be examined microscopically. Typically, pathologists section and evaluate 1 to 2 areas of a submitted specimen and full evaluation needs to be requested.[91,92] Similarly, incisional biopsy is not enough to diag-nose unicystic ameloblastoma or determine whether it is amenable to enucleation (ie, if only luminal/intraluminal ameloblastoma is found). Those with mural involvement should have resection.[89,93,94]

Future directions

Ameloblastoma requires highly invasive ablation and reconstruction. The ability to lessen surgical burden almost certainly lies with adjunctive or pri-mary medical therapy. The genetic abnormalities have recently been identified.[95] Using primary cell lines of ameloblastoma, Kurppa and col-leagues[96] showed that epidermal growth factor re-ceptors stopped proliferation of 1 of 2 lines. This finding prompted them to study downstream mu-tations and they identified mutations in BRAF, an oncogene within the MAP kinase pathway, in 63% of ameloblastoma samples. Another group then reported BRAF mutations in 46% of amelo-blastoma samples (predominantly mandibular le-sions) and found additional mutations in Smoothened (SMO) of the Sonic hedgehog pathway (predominantly maxillary lesions).[97] Sub-sequently, in a larger series (84 ameloblastomas), 88% had mutations in the MAP kinase pathway (62% BRAF).[98]

Mutations in these pathways are found in other neoplasms, such as melanoma and colorectal carcinoma, and effective inhibitors exist.[99,100] Sys-temic side effects of new inhibitors have limited utilization in the treatment of benign disease pro-cesses. Limited success has been reported for use of directed inhibitors to mutations identified in multiply recurrent or multifocal lesions.[101–104] It is hoped that additional formulations and/or routes of administration (eg, topical administration) can make routine use possible to lessen surgical morbidity.

SUMMARY

Benign maxillofacial lesions may not be life threat-ening, but treatment of these lesions can have a serious impact on the patients. Within the maxillo-facial region, the OKC, GCL, and ameloblastoma are common locally destructive benign entities with a tendency to recur. The development of less invasive procedures and treatment adjuncts has decreased the morbidity of treatment with reasonable outcomes. As more is understood about the molecular and genetic causes of these lesions, more directed medical therapy could lessen the burden of operative treatment.

REFERENCES

1. Shear M. The aggressive nature of the odontogenic keratocyst: is it a benign cystic neoplasm? Part 1. Clinical and early experimental evidence of aggressive behaviour. Oral Oncol 2002;38(3): 219–26.
2. Shear M. The aggressive nature of the odontogenic keratocyst: is it a benign cystic neoplasm? Part 2. Proliferation and genetic studies. Oral Oncol 2002;38(4):323–31.
3. Vedtofte P, Praetorius F. Recurrence of the odonto-genic keratocyst in relation to clinical and histolog-ical features. A 20-year follow-up study of 72 patients. Int J Oral Surg 1979;8(6):412–20.
4. Brannon RB. The odontogenic keratocyst. A clini-copathologic study of 312 cases. Part I. Clinical features. Oral Surg Oral Med Oral Pathol 1976; 42(1):54–72.
5. Rud J, Pindborg JJ. Odontogenic keratocysts: a follow-up study of 21 cases. J Oral Surg 1969; 27(5):323–30.
6. Bataineh AB, al Qudah M. Treatment of mandibular odontogenic keratocysts. Oral Surg Oral Med Oral Pathol Oral Radiol Endod 1998;86(1):42–7.
7. el-Hajj G, Anneroth G. Odontogenic keratocysts–a retrospective clinical and histologic study. Int J Oral Maxillofac Surg 1996;25(2):124–9.
8. Chuong R, Donoff RB, Guralnick W. The odonto-genic keratocyst. J Oral Maxillofac Surg 1982; 40(12):797–802.

9. Irvine GH, Bowerman JE. Mandibular keratocysts: surgical management. Br J Oral Maxillofac Surg 1985;23(3):204–9.

10. Stoelinga PJ. Long-term follow-up on keratocysts treated according to a defined protocol. Int J Oral Maxillofac Surg 2001;30(1):14–25.

11. Madras J, Lapointe H. Keratocystic odontogenic tumour: reclassification of the odontogenic keratocyst from cyst to tumour. J Can Dent Assoc 2008; 74(2):165-165h.

12. Forssell K, Forssell H, Kahnberg KE. Recurrence of keratocysts. A long-term follow-up study. Int J Oral Maxillofac Surg 1988;17(1):25–8.

13. Pogrel MA. The keratocystic odontogenic tumor. Oral Maxillofac Surg Clin North Am 2013;25(1): 21–30.

14. Kolokythas A, Fernandes RP, Pazoki A, et al. Odontogenic keratocyst: to decompress or not to decompress? A comparative study of decompression and enucleation versus resection/peripheral ostectomy. J Oral Maxillofac Surg 2007;65(4): 640–4.

15. Nakamura N, Mitsuyasu T, Mitsuyasu Y, et al. Marsupialization for odontogenic keratocysts: long-term follow-up analysis of the effects and changes in growth characteristics. Oral Surg Oral Med Oral Pathol Oral Radiol Endod 2002; 94(5):543–53.

16. Sharif FNj, Oliver R, Sweet C, et al. Interventions for the treatment of keratocystic odontogenic tumours (KCOT, odontogenic keratocysts (OKC)). Cochrane Database Syst Rev 2010;(9):CD008464.

17. Pogrel MA. The keratocystic odontogenic tumour (KCOT)–an odyssey. Int J Oral Maxillofac Surg 2015;44(12):1565–8.

18. Pogrel MA. The use of liquid nitrogen cryotherapy in the management of locally aggressive bone lesions. J Oral Maxillofac Surg 1993;51(3):269–73.

19. Schmidt BL, Pogrel MA. The use of enucleation and liquid nitrogen cryotherapy in the management of odontogenic keratocysts. J Oral Maxillofac Surg 2001;59(7):720–5.

20. Pogrel MA, Regezi JA, Fong B, et al. Effects of liquid nitrogen cryotherapy and bone grafting on artificial bone defects in minipigs: a preliminary study. Int J Oral Maxillofac Surg 2002;31(3): 296–302.

21. Schmidt BL, Pogrel MA. Neurosensory changes after liquid nitrogen cryotherapy. J Oral Maxillofac Surg 2004;62(10):1183–7.

22. Fisher AD, Williams DF, Bradley PF. The effect of cryosurgery on the strength of bone. Br J Oral Surg 1978;15(3):215–22.

23. Blanas N, Freund B, Schwartz M, et al. Systematic review of the treatment and prognosis of the odontogenic keratocyst. Oral Surg Oral Med Oral Pathol Oral Radiol Endod 2000;90(5):553–8.

24. Johnson NR, Batstone MD, Savage NW. Management and recurrence of keratocystic odontogenic tumor: a systematic review. Oral Surg Oral Med Oral Pathol Oral Radiol 2013;116(4): e271–6.

25. US Food and Drug Administration Section 460.200 FDA compliance policy guides. Washington, DC: Food and Drug Administration; 1992. p. 219.

26. Dashow JE, McHugh JB, Braun TM, et al. Significantly decreased recurrence rates in keratocystic odontogenic tumor with simple enucleation and curettage using Carnoy's Versus modified Carnoy's solution. J Oral Maxillofac Surg 2015;73(11): 2132–5.

27. Toller PA. Protein substances in odontogenic cyst fluids. Br Dent J 1970;128(7):317–22.

28. Toller PA. The osmolality of fluids from cysts of the jaws. Br Dent J 1970;129(6):275–8.

29. Pogrel MA, Jordan RC. Marsupialization as a definitive treatment for the odontogenic keratocyst. J Oral Maxillofac Surg 2004;62(6):651–5 [discussion: 655–6]. [Erratum appears in: J Oral Maxillofac Surg 2007;65(2):362–3].

30. Marker P, Brøndum N, Clausen PP, et al. Treatment of large odontogenic keratocysts by decompression and later cystectomy: a long-term follow-up and a histologic study of 23 cases. Oral Surg Oral Med Oral Pathol Oral Radiol Endod 1996; 82(2):122–31.

31. Brøndum N, Jensen VJ. Recurrence of keratocysts and decompression treatment. A long-term follow-up of forty-four cases. Oral Surg Oral Med Oral Pathol 1991;72(3):265–9.

32. August M, Faquin WC, Troulis MJ, et al. Dedifferentiation of odontogenic keratocyst epithelium after cyst decompression. J Oral Maxillofac Surg 2003; 61(6):678–83.

33. Wright JM, Vered M. Update from the 4th Edition of the World Health Organization classification of head and neck tumours: odontogenic and maxillofacial bone tumors. Head Neck Pathol 2017;11(1): 68–77.

34. Barreto DC, Gomez RS, Bale AE, et al. PTCH gene mutations in odontogenic keratocysts. J Dent Res 2000;79(6):1418–22.

35. Shimada Y, Katsube K, Kabasawa Y, et al. Integrated genotypic analysis of hedgehog-related genes identifies subgroups of keratocystic odontogenic tumor with distinct clinicopathological features. PLoS One 2013;8(8):e70995.

36. Qu J, Yu F, Hong Y, et al. Underestimated PTCH1 mutation rate in sporadic keratocystic odontogenic tumors. Oral Oncol 2015;51(1):40–5.

37. Sun LS, Li XF, Li TJ. PTCH1 and SMO gene alterations in keratocystic odontogenic tumors. J Dent Res 2008;87(6):575–9.

38. Rui Z, Li-Ying P, Jia-Fei Q, et al. Smoothened gene alterations in keratocystic odontogenic tumors. Head Face Med 2014;10:36.

39. Frampton JE, Basset-Séguin N. Vismodegib: a review in advanced basal cell carcinoma. Drugs 2018;78(11):1145–56.

40. Bergström D, Page DR, Rogers G, et al. Two intermittent vismodegib dosing regimens in patients with multiple basal-cell carcinomas (MIKIE): a randomised, regimen-controlled, double-blind, phase 2 trial. Lancet Oncol 2017;18(3):404–12.

41. Goldberg LH, Landau JM, Moody MN, et al. Resolution of odontogenic keratocysts of the jaw in basal cell nevus syndrome with GDC-0449. Arch Dermatol 2011;147(7):839–41.

42. Ally MS, Tang JY, Joseph T, et al. The use of vismodegib to shrink keratocystic odontogenic tumors in patients with basal cell nevus syndrome. JAMA Dermatol 2014;150(5):542–5.

43. Booms P, Harth M, Sader R, et al. Vismodegib hedgehog-signaling inhibition and treatment of basal cell carcinomas as well as keratocystic odontogenic tumors in Gorlin syndrome. Ann Maxillofac Surg 2015;5(1):14–9.

44. Ledderhof NJ, Caminiti MF, Bradley G, et al. Topical 5-fluorouracil is a novel targeted therapy for the keratocystic odontogenic tumor. J Oral Maxillofac Surg 2016;75(3):514–24.

45. Terry B, Jacoway J. Management of central giant cell lesions: an alternative to surgical therapy. Oral Maxillofac Surg Clin North Am 1994; 6:579.

46. Carlos R, Sedano HO. Intralesional corticosteroids as an alternative treatment for central giant cell granuloma. Oral Surg Oral Med Oral Pathol Oral Radiol Endod 2002;93:161.

47. Nogueira RL, Teixeira RC, Cavalcante RB, et al. Intralesional injection of triamcinolone hexacetonide as an alternative treatment for central giant-cell granuloma in 21 cases. Int J Oral Maxillofac Surg 2010;39:1204.

48. Harris M. Central giant cell granulomas of the jaws regress with calcitonin therapy. Br J Oral Maxillofac Surg 1993;31:89.

49. Pogrel MA. Calcitonin therapy for central giant cell granuloma. J Oral Maxillofac Surg 2003;61:649.

50. de Lange J, van den Akker HP, Veldhuijzen van Zanten GO, et al. Calcitonin therapy in central giant cell granuloma of the jaw: a randomized double-blind placebo-controlled study. Int J Oral Maxillofac Surg 2006;35:791.

51. Kaban LB, Mulliken JB, Ezekowitz RA, et al. Antiangiogenic therapy of a recurrent giant cell tumor of the mandible with interferon alfa-2a. Pediatrics 1999;103:1145.

52. Itonaga I, Hussein I, Kudo O, et al. Cellular mechanisms of osteoclast formation and lacunar resorption in giant cell granuloma of the jaw. J Oral Pathol Med 2003;32:224.

53. Flanagan AM, Nui B, Tinkler SM, et al. The multinucleate cells in giant cell granulomas of the jaw are osteoclasts. Cancer 1988;62:1139.

54. Chuong R, Kaban LB, Kozakewich H, et al. Central giant cell lesions of the jaws: a clinicopathologic study. J Oral Maxillofac Surg 1986;44:708.

55. Ficarra G, Kaban LB, Hansen LS. Central giant cell lesions of the mandible and maxilla: a clinicopathologic and cytometric study. Oral Surg Oral Med Oral Pathol 1987;64:44.

56. Schreuder WH, van den Berg H, Westermann AM, et al. Pharmacological and surgical therapy for the central giant cell granuloma: a long-term retrospective cohort study. J Craniomaxillofac Surg 2017;45(2):232–43.

57. Schreuder WH, Coumou AW, Kessler PA, et al. Alternative pharmacologic therapy for aggressive central giant cell granuloma: denosumab. J Oral Maxillofac Surg 2014;72:1301.

58. Schreuder WH, Peacock ZS, Ebb D, et al. Adjuvant antiangiogenic treatment for aggressive giant cell lesions of the jaw: a 20-year experience at Massachusetts General Hospital. J Oral Maxillofac Surg 2017;75(1):105–18.

59. Chawla S, Henshaw R, Seeger L, et al. Safety and efficacy of denosumab for adults and skeletally mature adolescents with giant cell tumour of bone: interim analysis of an open-label, parallel-group, phase 2 study. Lancet Oncol 2013;14:901.

60. Bredell M, Rordorf T, Kroiss S, et al. Denosumab as a treatment alternative for central giant cell granuloma: a long-term retrospective cohort study. J Oral Maxillofac Surg 2018;76(4):775–84.

61. Lipplaa A, Dijkstra S, Gelderblom H. Challenges of denosumab in giant cell tumor of bone, and other giant cell-rich tumors of bone. Curr Opin Oncol 2019;31(4):329–35.

62. Wang HD, Boyce AM, Tsai JY, et al. Effects of denosumab treatment and discontinuation on human growth plates. J Clin Endocrinol Metab 2014; 99(3):891–7.

63. Boyce AM, Chong WH, Yao J, et al. Denosumab treatment for fibrous dysplasia. J Bone Miner Res 2012;27(7):1462–70.

64. de Castro LF, Burke AB, Wang HD, et al. Activation of RANK/RANKL/OPG pathway is involved in the pathophysiology of fibrous dysplasia and associated with disease burden. J Bone Miner Res 2019;34(2):290–4.

65. Boquete-Castro A, Gómez-Moreno G, Calvo-Guirado JL, et al. Denosumab and osteonecrosis of the jaw. A systematic analysis of events reported in clinical trials. Clin Oral Implants Res 2016;27(3): 367–75.

66. Peacock ZS, Schwab JH, Faquin WC, et al. Genetic analysis of giant cell lesions of the maxillofacial and axial/appendicular skeletons. J Oral Maxillofac Surg 2017;75(2):298–308.

67. Presneau N, Baumhoer D, Behjati S, et al. Diagnostic value of H3F3A mutations in giant cell tumour of bone compared to osteoclast-rich mimics. J Pathol Clin Res 2015;1:113.

68. Gomes CC, Diniz MG, Amaral FR, et al. The highly prevalent H3F3A mutation in giant cell tumours of bone is not shared by sporadic central giant cell lesion of the jaws. Oral Surg Oral Med Oral Pathol Oral Radiol 2014;118:583.

69. Resnick CM, Margolis J, Susarla SM, et al. Maxillofacial and axial/appendicular giant cell lesions: unique tumors or variants of the same disease?–A comparison of phenotypic, clinical, and radiographic characteristics. J Oral Maxillofac Surg 2010;68:130.

70. Peacock ZS, Resnick CM, Susarla SM, et al. Do histologic criteria predict biologic behavior of giant cell lesions? J Oral Maxillofac Surg 2012;70:2573.

71. Antonoglou GN, Sandor GK. Recurrence rates of intraosseous ameloblastomas of the jaws: a systematic review of conservative versus aggressive treatment approaches and meta-analysis of non-randomized studies. J Craniomaxillofac Surg 2015;43:149.

72. Almeida RA, Andrade ES, Barbalho JC, et al. Recurrence rate following treatment for primary multicystic ameloblastoma: systematic review and meta-analysis. Int J Oral Maxillofac Surg 2016;45:359.

73. Reichart PA, Philipsen HP, Sonner S. Ameloblastoma: biological profile of 3677 cases. Eur J Cancer B Oral Oncol 1995;31B:86.

74. Sehdev MK, Huvos AG, Strong EW, et al. Ameloblastoma of maxilla and mandible. Cancer 1974;33:324.

75. Vedtofte P, Hjorting-Hansen E, Jensen BN, et al. Conservative surgical treatment of mandibular ameloblastomas. Int J Oral Surg 1978;7(3):156–61.

76. Huffman GG, Thatcher JW. Ameloblastoma–the conservative surgical approach to treatment: report of four cases. J Oral Surg 1974;32(11):850–4.

77. Sachs SA. Surgical excision with peripheral ostectomy: a definitive, yet conservative, approach to the surgical management of ameloblastoma. J Oral Maxillofac Surg 2006;64(3):476–83.

78. Mehlisch DR, Dahlin DC, Masson JK. Ameloblastoma: a clinicopathologic report. J Oral Surg 1972;30(1):9–22.

79. Nastri AL, Wiesenfeld D, Radden BG, et al. Maxillary ameloblastoma: a retrospective study of 13 cases. Br J Oral Maxillofac Surg 1995;33(1):28–32.

80. Oka K, Fukui M, Yamashita M, et al. Mandibular ameloblastoma with intracranial extension and distant metastasis. Clin Neurol Neurosurg 1986;88(4):303–9.

81. Hayward JR. Recurrent ameloblastoma 30 years after surgical treatment. J Oral Surg 1973;31(5):368–70.

82. Daramola JO, Ajagbe HA, Oluwasanmi JO. Recurrent ameloblastoma of the jaws–a review of 22 cases. Plast Reconstr Surg 1980;65(5):577–9.

83. Adekeye EO, Lavery KM. Recurrent ameloblastoma of the maxillo-facial region. Clinical features and treatment. J Maxillofac Surg 1986;14(3):153–7.

84. Robinson L, Martinez MG. Unicystic ameloblastoma: a prognostically distinct entity. Cancer 1977;40(5):2278–85.

85. Leider AS, Eversole LR, Barkin ME. Cystic ameloblastoma. A clinicopathologic analysis. Oral Surg Oral Med Oral Pathol 1985;60:624.

86. Li TJ, Wu YT, Yu SF, et al. Unicystic ameloblastoma: a clinicopathologic study of 33 Chinese patients. Am J Surg Pathol 2000;24:1385.

87. Wang JT. Unicystic ameloblastoma: a clinicopathological appraisal. Taiwan Yi Xue Hui Za Zhi 1985;84:1363.

88. Lau SL, Samman N. Recurrence related to treatment modalities of unicystic ameloblastoma: a systematic review. Int J Oral Maxillofac Surg 2006;35:681.

89. Chouinard AF, Peacock ZS, Faquin WC, et al. Unicystic ameloblastoma revisited: comparison of Massachusetts General Hospital outcomes with original Robinson and Martinez report. J Oral Maxillofac Surg 2017;75(11):2369–78.

90. Gardner DG, Corio RL. Plexiform unicystic ameloblastoma, a variant of ameloblastoma with a low-recurrence rate after enucleation. Cancer 1984;53:1730.

91. Kessler HP. Intraosseous ameloblastoma. Oral Maxillofac Surg Clin North Am 2004;16:309.

92. Guthrie D, Peacock ZS, Sadow P, et al. Preoperative incisional and intraoperative frozen section biopsy techniques have comparable accuracy in the diagnosis of benign intraosseous jaw pathology. J Oral Maxillofac Surg 2012;70:2566.

93. Gardner DG, Pecak AMJ. The treatment of ameloblastoma based on pathologic and anatomic principles. Cancer 1980;46:2514.

94. Feinberg SE, Steinberg B. Surgical management of ameloblastoma. Current status of the literature. Oral Surg Oral Med Oral Pathol Oral Radiol Endod 1996;81:383.

95. Gomes CC, Duarte AP, Diniz MG, et al. Review article: current concepts of ameloblastoma pathogenesis. J Oral Pathol Med 2010;39(8):585–91.

96. Kurppa KJ, Catón J, Morgan PR, et al. High frequency of BRAF V600E mutations in ameloblastoma. J Pathol 2014;232(5):492–8.

97. Sweeney RT, McClary AC, Myers BR, et al. Identification of recurrent SMO and BRAF mutations in ameloblastomas. Nat Genet 2014;46(7): 722–5.

98. Brown NA, Rolland D, McHugh JB, et al. Activating FGFR2-RAS-BRAF mutations in ameloblastoma. Clin Cancer Res 2014;20(21):5517–26.

99. Salama AK, Flaherty KT. BRAF in melanoma: current strategies and future directions. Clin Cancer Res 2013;19(16):4326–34.

100. Gong J, Cho M, Fakih M. RAS and BRAF in metastatic colorectal cancer management. J Gastrointest Oncol 2016;7(5):687–704.

101. Kaye FJ, Ivey AM, Drane WE, et al. Clinical and radiographic response with combined BRAF-targeted therapy in stage 4 ameloblastoma. J Natl Cancer Inst 2014;107(1):378.

102. Faden DL, Algazi A. Durable treatment of ameloblastoma with single agent BRAFi Re: clinical and radiographic response with combined BRAF-targeted therapy in stage 4 ameloblastoma. J Natl Cancer Inst 2016;109(1) [pii:djw190].

103. Tan S, Pollack JR, Kaplan MJ, et al. BRAF inhibitor therapy of primary ameloblastoma. Oral Surg Oral Med Oral Pathol Oral Radiol 2016;122(4):518–9.

104. Fernandes GS, Girardi DM, Bernardes JPG, et al. Clinical benefit and radiological response with BRAF inhibitor in a patient with recurrent ameloblastoma harboring V600E mutation. BMC Cancer 2018;18(1):887.

Current Methods of Maxillofacial Tissue Engineering

James C. Melville, DDS[a], Victoria A. Mañón, DDS[b], Caleb Blackburn, DDS[c], Simon Young, DDS, MD, PhD[b],*

KEYWORDS

- Tissue engineering • Platelet-rich plasma (PRP) • Platelet-rich fibrin (PRF)
- Bone marrow aspirate concentrate (BMAC) • Bone morphogenic protein (BMP)
- Composite allogeneic grafting

KEY POINTS

- With the advent of tissue engineering–based approaches, the embryonic process of tissue generation can be recapitulated using mesenchymal stem cells (MSCs), growth factors, and cytokines. These elements can be found in platelet-rich plasma (PRP), platelet-rich fibrin (PRF), bone morphogenic protein (BMP), and bone marrow aspirate concentrate (BMAC).
- Tissue engineering provides an alternative reconstructive modality that can decrease surgical morbidity and duration of inpatient hospitalization, while maintaining excellent postoperative outcomes and effective bone regeneration.
- Advances in tissue engineering research include the use of 3-dimensional printers for the fabrication of porous, flexible scaffolds, and new tissue engineering techniques for the regeneration of muscle, bone, and cartilage.
- This article explores the history, biological basis, and examples of applications of MSC, PRP, PRF, BMP, and BMAC, used individually and in combination for tissue engineering in oral and maxillofacial surgery.

INTRODUCTION TO TISSUE REGENERATION

In the early 1970s, W. T. Green, a pediatric orthopedic surgeon at Boston Children's Hospital, first introduced the concept of tissue engineering by undertaking several experiments aimed to generate cartilage from chondrocytes seeded in bone spicules.[1] Since then, several major research centers around the world have continued to explore and advance tissue engineering. In 1993, Drs Robert Langer and Joseph Vacanti described tissue engineering as "an interdisciplinary field that applies the principles of engineering and the life sciences toward the development of biological substitutes that restore, maintain, or improve tissue function."[2] The formation of the Tissue Engineering Regenerative Medicine International Society in 2003 highlighted a major milestone and has united scientists worldwide to share and collaborate on their research. These joint efforts have translated to significant improvements in the clinical setting by increasing efficiency and

Disclosure Statement: The authors have nothing to disclose.
[a] Oral, Head & Neck Oncology and Microvascular Reconstructive Surgery, Department of Oral and Maxillofacial Surgery, University of Texas Health Science Center, School of Dentistry, 6560 Fannin Street, Suite 1900, Houston, TX 77030, USA; [b] Department of Oral and Maxillofacial Surgery, University of Texas Health Science Center, School of Dentistry, 7500 Cambridge Street, Suite 6510, Houston, TX 77054, USA; [c] Department of Oral and Maxillofacial Surgery, University of Tennessee Medical Center, 1930 Alcoa Highway, Suite 335, Knoxville, TN 37920 USA
* Corresponding author.
E-mail address: Simon.Young@uth.tmc.edu

Oral Maxillofacial Surg Clin N Am 31 (2019) 579–591
https://doi.org/10.1016/j.coms.2019.07.003
1042-3699/19/© 2019 Elsevier Inc. All rights reserved.

postoperative outcome while decreasing patient morbidity and surgical complications.[3–5]

Despite the numerous materials used in tissue engineering, there are 3 essential factors required for successful regeneration: (1) scaffolding, or a framework for tissue regeneration, (2) cell signaling for the promotion of stem cell differentiation and cell migration, and (3) regenerative/stem cells (**Fig. 1**). **Table 1** gives a brief outline of previously used materials for each of these factors in maxillofacial bone tissue engineering approaches.

This review focuses on the use of allogeneic bone as the scaffold, recombinant human bone morphogenic protein-2 (rhBMP-2) and platelet-rich plasma (PRP)/platelet-rich fibrin (PRF) as the cell signaling molecules, and bone marrow aspirate concentrate (BMAC) as the source of mesenchymal stem cells (MSCs).

The reconstruction of maxillofacial defects is associated with many challenges, including an elevated risk of infection associated with the polymicrobial environment of the oral cavity and occasionally insufficient volume of the surrounding soft tissue envelope. Mandibular continuity defects often result from resection of tumors or trauma. Traditionally, the gold standard for reconstruction includes the use of autogenous bone or osteocutaneous free flaps.[15] Vascularized free flaps require a donor site, posing an additional risk for complications, and greatly increase morbidity for the patient. These procedures require a longer length of hospital stay, more involved wound care, and rehabilitation of the donor limb with physical therapy.[15]

Despite their traditional use, autogenous bone grafts are not without risks either. They often result in multiple, staged surgeries and carry the risk of nerve damage and scarring. Because of the elevated risk of bacterial contamination from the oral cavity, when an autogenous bone graft is treatment planned, many surgeons elect to complete

Table 1
Previously used materials in maxillofacial bone tissue engineering approaches

Approach	Materials
Scaffolds[3–9]	Natural polymers (collagen) Synthetic polymers, including: • Polylactic acid (PLA) • Polyglycolic acid (PGA) • Copolymers of PLA and PGA [poly(DL- lactic-co-glycolic acid)] • Polycaprolacedittones Calcium phosphate ceramics • Hydroxyapatite • Tricalcium phosphate • Beta tricalcium phosphate Xenogeneic bone Allogeneic bone
Cell Signaling[3,10–12]	Bone morphogenic proteins (BMP-2 and -7) Platelet-rich plasma Platelet-rich fibrin Mechanical bioreactors
Regenerative Cells[3,13–15]	Dental tissue–derived mesenchymal stem cells (MSCs) • Dental pulp stem cells • Periodontal ligament stem cells • Stem cells from human exfoliated deciduous teeth • Stem cells from apical papilla • Dental follicle progenitor cells Periosteal-derived cells Adipose-derived stem cells Bone marrow MSCs

the reconstruction during a second-stage surgery to allow for complete intraoral healing of the primary resection. In addition, they often elect a transcervical surgical approach that comes with the risk of nerve injury and unaesthetic scarring.

With the advent of tissue engineering–based approaches, the embryonic process of tissue generation can be recapitulated using MSCs, growth factors, and cytokines. These elements can be found in PRP, PRF, BMP, and BMAC. This article explores their history, biological basis, and examples of applications in oral and maxillofacial surgery. Tissue engineering provides an alternative

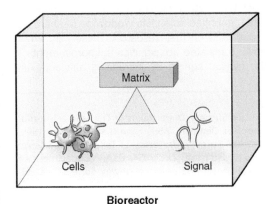

Bioreactor

Fig. 1. The classic tissue engineering triangle needed for bone regeneration.

reconstructive modality that can decrease surgical morbidity and duration of inpatient hospitalization, while maintaining excellent postoperative outcomes and effective bone regeneration.[13–15]

PLATELET-RICH PLASMA

In the 1970s, hematologists coined the concept of PRP, describing it as plasma with a platelet count higher than that of peripheral blood.[16,17] For the enhancement of hard and soft tissue wound healing, it has been suggested that a therapeutic dose of 1,000,000 platelets per microliter is necessary, as compared with the normal human blood range of 150,000 to 300,000 per microliter.[18–20] Initially used to treat patients with thrombocytopenia, oral and maxillofacial surgeons began to use it approximately 10 years later for its antiinflammatory properties in healing surgical wounds.[17,21] Used in combination with autogenous or allogeneic grafting materials, oral and maxillofacial surgeons have achieved predictable surgical outcomes. Other medical specialties, including orthopedic, cardiovascular, and plastic surgery also use PRP for its applications in tissue regeneration, wound healing, and scar revision.

Although the exact mechanisms of action and cellular pathways are complex and require further study, the wound healing properties of PRP result from the activation and degranulation of platelets, followed by the subsequent release of factors that promote angiogenesis, wound healing, tissue repair, and stem cell activity. Storage granules released from platelets include "alpha" and "delta" (also called "dense") granules, which contain polypeptides and small molecules, respectively, that actively recruit factors and cells to the site of injury.[22] Alpha granules contain various growth factors and proteins, including von Willebrand factor, fibrinogen, platelet-derived growth factor (PDGF), epithelial growth factor (EGF), vascular endothelial growth factor (VEGF), endothelial cell growth factor, fibroblast growth factor, transforming growth factor beta (TGF-β), and insulin-like growth factor (IGF). These factors function to activate stem cells, subsequently inducing chemotaxis, mitogenesis, and differentiation of other cells. Dense granules contain adenosine diphosphate/adenosine tri-phosphate, calcium, and serotonin; these function to increase vascular permeability and perfusion of the tissues. These factors act directly and cross-communicate to induce tissue regeneration, including amplification of the signaling effect of rhBMP-2/ acellular collagen sponge (ACS).[20,22]

PRP is a double-centrifuged preparation of a blood sample collected from the patient (**Fig. 2**).

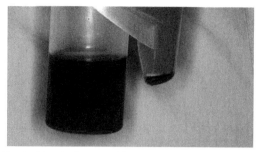

Fig. 2. Blood after centrifuging, separating the erythrocyte, plasma, and PRP.

The collected blood, ranging from 40 cc for minor procedures to 500 cc for larger reconstructions, is placed into a tube with an anticoagulant. The first spin separates the erythrocyte layer from the plasma, which contains the platelets and white blood cells (also known as the buffy coat). The erythrocytes are removed, and the tube is more lightly centrifuged again to delicately separate the PRP from the platelet poor plasma. This process concentrates the platelets in the blood by approximately 4 to 7 times.[19,23] The PRP can be stored up to 8 hours and must be activated before use by adding 5 mL of 10% calcium chloride with 5000 units of topical bovine thrombin.[24]

The risks associated with use of PRP are inherently low due to autogenous grafting, and the contraction of infectious diseases or immunogenic reactions associated with allogeneic or xenografts are eliminated. Risks associated with the use of bovine thrombin include the generation of antibodies to factors V and XI, resulting in coagulopathies associated with factor V deficiency.[24] In addition, variability in handling results in different PRP mixtures. Alteration of factors that increase variability include (1) centrifugation parameters, including speed and time, (2) and temperature. According to Amable and colleagues,[25] the most optimal results were obtained while centrifuging at 300 g for 5 minutes at 12°C or 240 g for 8 minutes at 16°C for the first spin and 700 g for 17 minutes at 12°C for the second spin.[23] Low temperature setting shave shown to delay platelet activation and prolong their viability. Despite positive results, differences in handling may account for variability of results found in the literature.[23]

PLATELET-RICH FIBRIN

Choukron and colleagues was one of the first researchers to describe PRF.[14,26] PRF is a second-generation autologous platelet concentration that has low cost and is relatively simple to process.[14] PRF is simpler than PRP to prepare in that no additional anticoagulants are added to the patient's peripheral blood.[27] In addition, one of the major advantages of PRF, sometimes referred to as leukocyte PRF (L-PRF), is having immune-compatible growth factors without the need of added bovine thrombin or other gelling agents.[14,27] Researchers have found that PRF contains a high concentration of bioactive growth factors that enhance wound healing through amplified chemotaxis, proliferation, differentiation, and angiogenesis.[14,27,28]

PRF consists of a fibrin matrix and several cells types and cellular products, such as platelets, leukocytes, cytokines, and circulating stem cells.[14,29] During centrifugation, the PRF clot is formed by a natural polymerization process. This natural process and subsequent fibrin architecture is responsible for the slow release of growth factors for 7 or more days.[14] PRF releases TGF-β, VEGF, PDGF-AB, and several glycoproteins, including thrombospondin-1, fibronectin, and vitronectin.[27] In addition to the growth factors released, recent studies have shown that the fibrin network itself has a major role in wound healing.[30] Leukocytes are highly important immune cells capable of directing and recruiting cell types during wound healing and participate in angiogenesis and lymphogenesis. Leukocytes promote later stages of wound healing while the fibrin network plays a role in the early stages of wound healing and these cells act synergistically with platelets, functioning as a reservoir of cytokines and the other glycoproteins previously mentioned.[30,31]

Many modifications of the protocols used for preparation of PRF have been described.[14,27,28,32] The main differences between the protocols are the centrifugation G-force and the centrifugation time. Standard PRF is traditionally done at 2700 revolutions per minute (rpm) for 12 minutes. Newer protocols, coined advanced PRF (A-PRF), reduce the revolutions to 1300 to 1500 rpm and increase the spin time to 14 minutes.[32] Choukroun and colleagues observed that reducing the centrifugation force led to increased total leukocyte numbers within PRF matrix scaffolds in A-PRF.[27] In addition, compared with L-PRF, A-PRF released significantly more growth factors, including PDGF, TGF- β1, VEGF, EGF, and IGF.

The physical and biological properties of PRF make it advantageous in several oral and maxillofacial surgery settings. Two such settings include PRF in particulate grafting procedures and as a palatal bandage for connective tissue graft donor sites.[33] PRF can be used to enhance the handling characteristics of a particulate bone graft. This is accomplished by hydrating particulate graft with the PRF membrane supernatant, creating a putty-like consistency.[14] Creation of PRF bone

putty incorporates the biological enhancement of wound healing, as well as increases the physical properties that make particulate bone easier to handle. The PRF bone putty is advantageous in socket graft applications and in lateral ridge augmentations.[14] Even with PRF alone, Alzahrani and colleagues showed that the use of PRF accelerates socket wound healing, demonstrated by radiographic and clinical bone fill.[34]

PRF can also be used as a palatal bandage for connective tissue graft donor sites. Common problems faced during connective tissue graft procedures is donor site bleeding, pain, and discomfort.[35] Epithelial cell migration and microvascularization are promoted by PRF, which makes it effective as a bandage for connective tissue graft donor sites. PRF when used as a palatal bandage reduces postoperative morbidity and significantly accelerates wound healing.[35,36] Additional applications for PRF membranes include coverage of implant surgical sites (**Fig. 3**C–E), bone-grafted sites (**Fig. 3**F–J), and areas of gingival recession.[37] PRF has also been shown to enhance implant stability after placement.[38] Oncu and colleagues observed that when PRF application was used during implant placement, the implant stability quotient was higher than the non-PRF group in the first weeks after surgery.[38]

In summary, PRF is a second-generation platelet concentrate that is both simple to process and inexpensive. The high amounts of growth factors found within PRF enhance wound healing through enhanced proliferation, chemotaxis, differentiation, and angiogenesis. The applications of PRF in the context of oral and maxillofacial surgery have the potential to increase the rate of wound healing and decrease patient morbidity.

BONE MORPHOGENIC PROTEIN

Another popular biologic used for maxillofacial tissue engineering is rhBMP-2. Part of the TGF-β superfamily, BMPs are one of the leading osteoinductive growth factors.[39] BMP promotes new bone formation by acting on cells at all stages of osteogenesis, from MSCs to mature osteocytes. Specifically, BMP-2 upregulates VEGF-A and promotes the differentiation of MSCs into osteoblasts.[40] BMP's activity was first described by Urist and has been studied since the 1960s but its popularity picked up in the 2000s.[39,41] In 2007 the use of rhBMP-2 was approved by the US Food and Drug Administration (FDA) for two maxillofacial surgical procedures: (1) localized alveolar ridge augmentation for defects associated with dental extractions and (2) maxillary sinus floor augmentation[s].[42] Histologic volume and quality

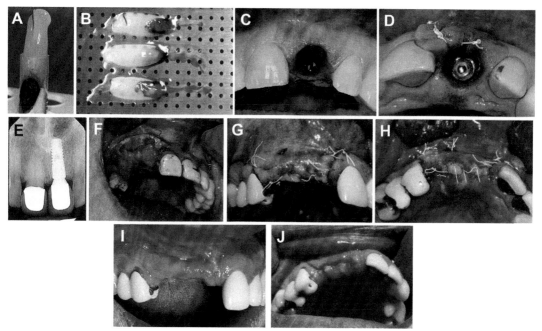

Fig. 3. (*A*) PRF clot removed from tube. (*B*) PRF clots on compression box. (*C*) Traumatic avulsion of tooth #9 treated with immediate implant placement and PRF bandage. (*D*) The PRF bandage placed on the facial alveolar surface. (*E*) Periapical radiograph of implant with provisional crown taken 3 months postoperatively. (*F*) Treatment of maxillary bony defect with cadaveric bone, PRP, and PRF. (*G, H*) Edentulous ridge immediately after closure when grafted with cadaveric bone, PRP, and PRF. (*I, J*) Edentulous ridge with adequate bone height and width for dental implant placement after healing from ridge augmentation with cadaveric bone, PRP, and PRF. (*Courtesy of* [*C, D, F–J*] Jonathon S. Jundt, DDS, MD, FACS, Houston, TX; and [*E*] Dr. Seung H. Lee, DDS, MS, Aurora, CO.)

of bone induced by rhBMP-2 at 6- and 12- month periods are found to be similar to the gold standard autogenous graft.[43]

Since BMP has been increasingly accepted in oral and maxillofacial surgery and is utilized in many other ways, it is important to explain to the patient that any other use of BMP is off-label and a proper consent should be obtained.[44,45] The FDA states that the contraindications to using rhBMP-2 in patients include: (1) allergic reaction to any of the materials contained in the devices, (2) active infection near the area of the surgical incision, (3) have had a tumor removed from the area of the implantation site or currently have a tumor in that area, (4) are skeletally immature, or (5) are pregnant. There are no definitive guidelines involving pediatric populations, so in general, caution should be exercised in patients less than 18-year-old.[46] In addition, clinicians should be cautious using BMP-2 in patients who are nursing and a negative pregnancy test should be obtained before performing the procedure.[47]

Several manufacturers produce rhBMP-2 and have made handling the product straight forward. The rhBMP-2 comes packaged as a lyophilized powder that can be reconstituted with prepackaged sterile water. This rhBMP-2 solution is then applied to an ACS. The ACS serves as both carrier for the protein and a scaffold for new bone formation. The patient should be forewarned that rhBMP-2 is associated with significant swelling and be aware of the risk for its use in surgery. This edema is attributed to the strong inflammatory cytokine-like properties of rhBMP-2 which induces mesenchymal stem cell differentiation.[15] It's important to note that a tension-free closure over the graft reduces the chances of wound dehiscence secondary to increasing postoperative edema.[47]

Apart from augmentation of the alveolar ridge and maxillary sinus floor, Herford and colleagues had successful outcomes when using BMP-2 in premaxillary cleft patients.[48] They demonstrated that using BMP alone in cleft patients yielded similar results to those patients grafted with the conventional approach of autogenous anterior iliac crest bone. The major benefit of this approach is the reduced need for a donor site and therefore theoretically decreased post-operative complications associated with such. In addition, Melville and colleagues demonstrated that BMP can be added to allogeneic bone grafts and bone marrow aspirate concentrate (BMAC) for immediate reconstruction of large mandibular defects with excellent outcomes.[15] BMP is also used in a variety of neurosurgical and orthopedic surgical procedures, including in acute open tibial fractures and anterior lumbar interbody spine fusion.[49]

In conclusion, recombinant human bone morphogenic protein-2 is a member of the transforming growth factor-beta superfamily with strong osteoinductive effects. rhBMP-2 promotes differentiation of MSCs into osteoblasts. The bone formation secondary to grafts using rhBMP-2 is similar to that of the gold-standard anterior iliac crest bone graft. rhBMP-2 is relatively easy to use and decreases the patient morbidity associated with a donor site. Although this recombinant growth factor is FDA approved for localized alveolar ridge augmentation for defects associated with dental extractions and maxillary sinus floor augmentation, several studies have shown the successful off-label use of rhBMP-2 in the reconstruction of large mandibular defects and alveolar clefts.

BONE MARROW ASPIRATE CONCENTRATE

Initially described in 1952, BMAC was first studied and used in various orthopedic procedures.[50] Also used to treat hematopoietic and oncologic diseases, BMAC was found to have additional uses as a cell source in the regeneration of other tissues in the body.[51] Although a traditional bone harvest does possess the cellular components necessary for bone regeneration, Marx and Harrell found that by concentrating the bone-forming cells, or the MSCs, and other necessary cellular components, osteogenesis and angiogenesis were optimized in the bone-forming process.[10] Bone marrow aspirate serves as a rich and readily available source of MSCs; MSCs have been demonstrated to be involved in both soft and hard tissue regeneration via paracrine cellular communication and contact between osteoblasts and progenitor stem cells. Of these cells, Marx and Harrell suggested that of the mixed cell population, CD34+, CD44+, CD90+, and CD105+ cells are the main types of osteoprogenitor cells found in the aspirate.[10] In addition, BMAC is rich in cytokines and growth factors that contribute to tissue regeneration.[51] Cassano and colleagues found that BMAC, as compared with PRP, has 172.5x the concentration of VEGF, 78x the concentration of interleukin 8 (IL-8), 4.6x the concentration of IL-1β, 3.4x the concentration of TGF-β2, and 1.3x the concentration of PDGF.[50,52] These multicellular interactions assist in tissue growth and development. Given these regenerative properties, it has since become widely popular among maxillofacial reconstructive surgeons because the aspiration procedure provides a treatment option that is relatively fast and simple with minimal morbidity to the patient (**Fig. 4**).

Several studies have shown that bone marrow derived stem and progenitor cells to be capable of regenerating bone in both animal and human models. Of the cleft lip and palate patients undergoing alveolar cleft lip repair, Gimbel and colleagues evaluated 69 patients divided into 3 groups: (1) grafting with bone marrow aspirate (BMA, aspirate without the concentration procedure) seeded onto a resorbable collagen matrix, (2) autogenous cortical and cancellous bone harvested from the ilium through a traditional open approach, and (3) autogenous cancellous bone that was collected from the ilium with a cannula.[53]

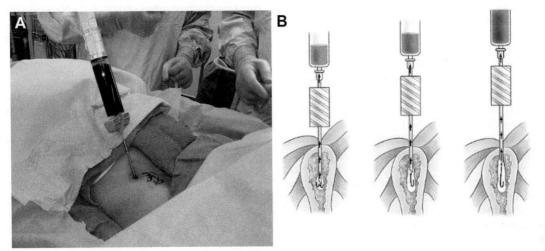

Fig. 4. (*A*) Harvest of BMAC with needle puncture through anterior ileum. (*B*) The steps of sequential bone marrow harvesting.

Although bone regeneration was comparable in all 3 groups, the patients in the BMA group experienced significantly less morbidity, operative time, and duration of hospital stay and cost. Of Melville and colleagues' patients who had undergone mandibular reconstruction using BMAC, BMP, and allogeneic bone for reconstruction, the success rate of the 5 patients was 100%, with all patients showing excellent bone quality clinically and radiographic dimensional adequacy for endosseous dental implant placement.[15] Their average postoperative hospital stay for the 5 patients was 2 days 12 hours, an improvement compared with the average postoperative hospital stay for more invasive reconstructive options.

Approved by the US FDA, BMAC can be obtained from the tibia, or anterior or posterior iliac crests, to deliver the patient's own MSCs to the defect site. A BMAC kit consists of a trocar, aspiration needle with syringe, and anticoagulant solution.[54] For each donor site, up to 120 cc of bone marrow aspirate can be obtained. Patient age must be accounted for, as the total number of viable mesenchymal cells has been found to be inversely proportional to age. If more bone marrow volume is needed, it is recommended to make a separate stab incision for additional harvest sites. In addition, this process can be repeated on the opposite ilium or tibia. Once collected, only 0.001% to 0.01% of all nucleated cells in the BMAC are MSCs, thus requiring a dual centrifugation process to further increase its concentration.[55] Once processed, the buffy coat layer and platelet poor plasma are removed; the remaining red blood cells layers are combined and centrifuged for a second time, separating the BMAC and the white cell pellet (**Fig. 5**). A hemanalysis with complete blood count is performed and recorded before injection.[54]

Contraindications to BMAC harvest include (1) bone diseases including congenital disorders (osteogenesis imperfecta), metabolic (osteopetrosis), or malignancy (multiple myeloma) or (2) history of radiation to the harvest site. Caution must be used when there is known anatomic deformity or history of trauma.[54]

COMPOSITE ALLOGENEIC TISSUE ENGINEERING

Although each of these factors has been used independently to assist in the regeneration of tissue, a composite allogeneic approach, or use of these factors in combination, has also shown to produce successful and predictable surgical outcomes. Various combinations of materials have been used over the years by multiple teams with

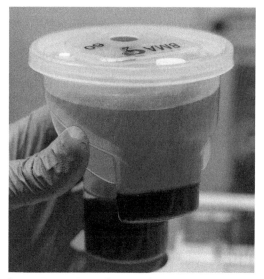

Fig. 5. Separation of mesenchymal stem cells from erythrocytes and plasma.

varying degrees of success. In 2001, Moghadam and colleagues combined poloxamer-based gel and human BMP to successfully regenerate bone in situ to reconstruct a 6 cm mandibular defect.[56–58] From 2004 to 2006, Warnke and colleagues used the latissimus dorsi of 3 patients to develop a replacement, customized vascularized mandible, and transplanted them into the respective patients to reconstruct up to 7 cm defects.[56,59] Melville and colleagues found that of the 5 patients who underwent mandibular reconstruction using BMAC, allogeneic bone, and rhBMP-2, all had successful outcomes resulting in excellent bone quality, clinically and radiographically, for dental rehabilitation using dental implants (**Fig. 6**).[15] Other studies have focused on the use of PRP/PRF in combination with other biomaterials. Kim and colleagues found that bone defects implanted with hydrogels impregnated with PRP, adipose, or

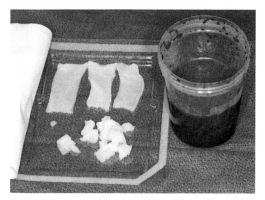

Fig. 6. BMAC + BMP + allogeneic bone.

bone marrow–derived stem cells exhibited strong differentiation potential toward osteogenic and chondrogenic regeneration.[60,61]

Although successful for the regeneration of bone, these techniques only allowed for the regeneration of homogeneous structures, such as bone, and do not allow for the regeneration of heterogeneous structures, such as joints, composed of bone and cartilage.[59] Tissue engineering can be used in combination with avascular grafts (**Figs. 7** and **8**) and vascular free flaps (**Fig. 9**) to reconstruct defects involving multiple tissues, to reduce patient morbidity associated with additional bone grafting sites, and to overcome problems associated with traditional grafting methods. In order to reconstruct the temporomandibular joint (TMJ) and mandibular body after resection of a unicystic ameloblastoma, Johnson and colleagues were able to regenerate sufficient mandibular bone height and width and reconstruct the condyle through the use of tissue engineering and costochondral rib grafting. The team used a resorbable mesh (poly-[D,L]-lactide copolymer), 120 mL of allogeneic corticocancellous bone, 12 mg of BMP, and 100 mL of BMAC, and the costochondral graft.[62] The patient achieved sufficient bone height and width for dental rehabilitation with endosseous implants without compromise of facial form or function and without the morbidity of an additional harvest to reconstruct the mandibular body. Melville and colleagues also used the combination of tissue engineering and a radial forearm flap to reconstruct a maxillary alveolar defect.[63] The extensive, posttraumatic maxillary defect did not have adequate soft tissue

coverage to successfully support a block graft. In addition, the radial forearm flap is reserved for small- to moderate-volume bony defects, as it is typically recommended that only 30% of the radius' cross-sectional area be harvested to avoid postoperative fracture; this lack of bulk is not ideal for the placement of dental implants and is not typically the first-choice treatment of maxillary reconstructions. In combination with the tissue engineering, this technique allowed for the supplementation of deficient, scarred gingival tissue and the reconstruction of the extensive defect in a manner conducive to future restoration. In order to overcome mandible fibula height discrepancies and altered interarch ridge relationships, Kim and colleagues proposed a novel technique using the superior border fibula placement with inferior grafting, incorporating virtual surgical planning and tissue engineering. They found that the technique allowed for a single-stage surgery with immediate implant placement; achieved favorable prosthetic and cosmetic outcomes for a large segmental mandibular defect (>9 cm); and that tissue engineering with BMP, PRP, and allogeneic bone can be safely used with a vascularized free flap.[64]

Despite these advances and growing body of literature, at this time there are no standardized protocols for tissue regeneration. Variations in the materials used, preparations, patient selection, and delivery method reduce the practitioner's ability to compare and reproduce findings. Nonetheless, the in situ tissue engineering strategy combining BMAC, BMP, and allogeneic bone graft is a promising approach for the reconstruction of large mandibular defects.

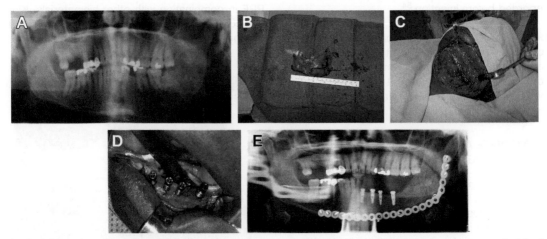

Fig. 7. (*A*) Panorex of large ossifying fibroma of the left mandible. (*B*) Resection of tumor via transcervical incision. (*C*) Placement of mixture BMAC + BMP + allogeneic graft into defect. (*D*) Dental implants placed 8 months post-op. (*E*) Panorex of dental implants after uncovering. Patient ready for dental prosthesis.

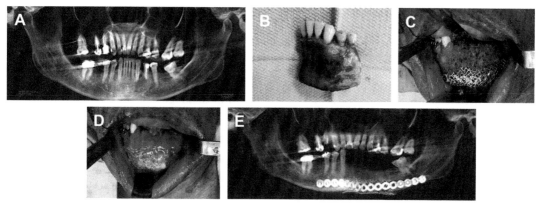

Fig. 8. (*A*) Panorex of ameloblastoma of the anterior mandible. (*B*) Resection of Anterior mandible via transoral approach. (*C*) Placement of BMAC + BMP + Allogeneic bone via transoral approach. (*D*) Strategic placement of BMP sponge soaked with BMAC placed under incision line to act as a membrane and aid in mucosal healing. Placement of stem cell poor plasma on to the rest of the graft as a biological membrane. (*E*) Panorex at 10 months post-op demonstrating well-consolidated bone graft ready for dental implant placement.

FUTURE APPLICATIONS

Tissue engineering is a continuously evolving area of interest and research. New developments are constantly occurring in areas of particular relevance to oral and maxillofacial surgery such as bone, muscle, and cartilage regeneration. For example, traditional bone grafting materials are often brittle, lack optimized porosity, and cannot easily be tailored to the specific needs of the patient.[65] Advances in 3-dimensional (3D) printing now allow the fabrication of bone regeneration scaffolds made to fit the specific functional and morphologic demands of the area of interest.[65–67] Fahimipour and colleagues conducted studies on 3D printed tricalcium phosphate–based scaffolds that were loaded with VEGF. These scaffolds were biomimetic porous scaffolds that slowly released VEGF, which promoted osteogenesis throughout the scaffold and proved to be a

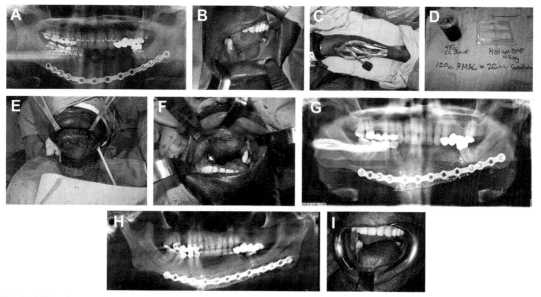

Fig. 9. (*A*) Patient presents status post mandibular resection of ameloblastoma reconstructed only with titanium reconstruction plate. (*B*) Intraoral soft tissue defect requiring soft tissue flap before bone graft. (*C*) Radial forearm flap for addition of soft tissue to the defect site. (*D*) BMAC + BMP + allogeneic bone. (*E*) Placement of tissue-engineered graft into defect. (*F*) Radial forearm flap in position within the oral cavity covering the defect. (*G*) Panorex of immediate bone graft. (*H*) Panorex at 8 months post-op demonstrating well-consolidated bone graft ready for implants. (*I*) Well-healed radial forearm flap covering mature bone graft.

potential treatment strategy for critical-sized bone defects.[68] In a related approach, Cui and colleagues used 3D printing to construct complex "biphasic" vascularized bone constructs.[69] These biphasic constructs were created using a dual bioprinting platform, generating a hard mineral structure surrounded by a soft organic matrix. The researchers then added BMP-2 and VEGF into the scaffolds to enhance osteogenesis and angiogenesis. This project was a proof of concept that mimicked native bone with high mechanical strength and a vascular network that is highly flexible.[69]

Aside from 3D printing materials with customized morphology, scaffolds can also be fabricated with surface characteristics similar to native extracellular matrix (ECM), yielding materials that allow for enhanced cell adhesion, proliferation, and differentiation. In the area of muscle regeneration, several groups are developing biomaterials that can present chemical and physical cues to muscle cells by mimicking the natural process of regeneration.[70,71] Examples include scaffolds aimed at mimicking the ECM of muscle fibers, which have been designed with myoinductive potential, that is, the ability to support growing muscle cells.[72] By adding cellular components and exogenous growth factors to these myoinductive scaffolds, researchers aim to optimize the body's ability to repair volumetric muscle loss.[72]

Lastly, others such as the Athanasiou Group have characterized tissues and studied various engineering techniques such as cell seeding, electrospinning, and self-assembling scaffold approaches to regenerate condylar cartilage and the TMJ disc.[73]

SUMMARY

In summary, tissue engineering has been studied for more than 30 years and continues to prove useful in oral and maxillofacial surgery. Early research in the field examined cartilage formation from bone spicules and low-cost fibrin matrices that aid in healing. Since then, tissue engineering in oral and maxillofacial surgery had advanced to the reconstruction of large craniomaxillofacial defects. From an office-based outpatient setting, BMP, PRF, and PRP can be easily added to the armamentarium, whereas BMAC is generally reserved for procedures under general anesthesia. Although the FDA has approved several techniques for dentoalveolar surgery, these protocols are being applied to reconstruct large segmental and critical-size maxillomandibular defects, as well. Three-dimensional printing has allowed researchers to print custom made, biomimetic scaffolds designed to treat the exact defect criteria in a patient-specific fashion. In conclusion, the advances of tissue engineering in oral and maxillofacial surgery have allowed for continual progress and improvement, as more research is devoted to reducing patient morbidity and improving the quality of life for patients.

REFERENCES

1. Vacanti CA. The history of tissue engineering. J Cell Mol Med 2006;10(3):569–76.
2. Langer R, Vacanti J. Tissue engineering. Science 1993;260:920.
3. Hutmacher DW. Scaffolds in tissue engineering bone and carti-lage. Biomaterials 2000;21:2529.
4. Bonzani IC, George JH, Stevens MM. Novel materials for bone and cartilage regeneration. Curr Opin Chem Biol 2006;10:568.
5. Williams JM, Adewunmi A, Schek RM, et al. Bone tissue engi- neering using polycaprolactone scaffolds fabricated via selective laser sintering. Biomaterials 2005;26:4817.
6. Yoshimoto H, Shin YM, Terai H, et al. A biodegradable nanofiber scaffold by electrospinning and its potential for bone tissue engineering. Biomaterials 2003;24: 2077.
7. Causa F, Netti PA, Ambrosio L, et al. Poly-epsilon-caprolactone/hydroxyapatite composites for bone regeneration: In vitro characterization and human osteoblast response. J Biomed Mater Res A 2006; 76:151.
8. Kweon H, Yoo MK, Park IK, et al. A novel degradable polycaprolactone networks for tissue engineering. Biomaterials 2003;24:801.
9. Cao T, Ho KH, Teoh SH. Scaffold design and in vitro study of osteochondral co-culture in a three-dimensional porous polycaprolactone scaffold fabricated by fused deposition modeling. Tissue Eng 2003;9(suppl 1):S103.
10. Marx RE, Harrell DB. Translational research: the CD34+ cell is crucial for large-volume bone regeneration from the milieu of bone marrow progenitor cells in craniomandibular reconstruction. Oral Craniofac Tissue Eng 2012;2(4):e201–9.
11. Herford AS, Boyne PJ. Reconstruction of mandibular continuity defects with bone morphogenetic protein-2 (rhBMP-2). J Oral Maxillofac Surg 2008;66:616.
12. Hoffmann A, Gross G. BMP signaling pathways in cartilage and bone formation. Crit Rev Eukaryot Gene Expr 2001;11:23.
13. Jäger M, Herten M, Fochtmann U, et al. Bridging the gap: bone marrow aspiration concentrate reduces autologous bone grafting in osseous defects. J Orthop Res 2011;29(2):173–80.
14. Melville JC, Shum JW, Young S, et al. Regenerative strategies for maxillary and mandibular

reconstruction: a practical guide. Springer International Publishing; 2019. Available at: www.springer.com/us/book/9783319936673.

15. Melville JC, Nassari NN, Hanna IA, et al. Immediate transoral allogeneic bone grafting for large mandibular defects. Less morbidity, more bone. A paradigm in benign tumor mandibular reconstruction? J Oral Maxillofac Surg 2016;75(4):828–38.

16. Andia I, Abate M. Platelet rich plasma: underlying biology and clinical correlates. Regen Med 2013;8: 645–58.

17. Andia I. Platelet-rich plasma biology. In: Alves R, Grimalt R, editors. Clinical indications and treatment protocols with platelet-rich plasma in dermatology. Barcelona (Spain): Ediciones Mayo; 2016. p. 3–15.

18. Marx RE, Carlson ER, Eichstaedt RM, et al. Platelet-rich plasma: growth factor enhancement for bone grafts. Oral Surg Oral Med Oral Pathol Oral Radiol Endod 1998;85:638–46.

19. Liao H-T, Marra KG, Rubin JP. Application of platelet-rich plasma and platelet-rich fibrin in fat grafting: basic science and literature review. Tissue Eng B Rev 2014;20:267–76.

20. Marx RE. Platelet-rich plasma: evidence to support its use. J Oral Maxillofac Surg 2004;62(4):489–96.

21. Alves R, Grimalt R. A review of platelet-rich plasma: history, biology, mechanism of action, and classification. Skin Appendage Disord 2017;4(1):18–24.

22. Sanchez-Gonzalez DJ, Mendez-Bolaina E, Trejo'-Bahena NI. Platelet-rich plasma peptides: key for regeneration. Int J Pept 2012;2012:532519.

23. Perez AGM, Lana JFSD, Rodrigues AA, et al. Relevant aspects of centrifugation step in the preparation of platelet rich plasma. ISRN Hematol 2014; 2014:176060.

24. Choi J, Minn KW, Chang H. The efficacy and safety of platelet-rich plasma and adipose-derived stem cells: an update. Arch Plast Surg 2012;39(6): 585–92.

25. Amable PR, Carias RBV, Teixeira MVT, et al. Platelet-rich plasma preparation for regenerative medicine: optimization and quantification of cytokines and growth factors. Stem Cell Res Ther 2013;4:67.

26. Choukroun J, Adda F, Schoeffer C, et al. PRF: "An opportunity in perioimplantology." Implantodontie 2000;42:55.

27. Choukroun J, Ghanaati S. Reduction of relative centrifugation force within injectable Platelet-Rich-Fibrin (PRF) Concentrates Advances Patients' Own Inflammatory Cells, Platelets and Growth Factors: The First Introduction to the Low Speed Centrifugation Concept. Eur J Trauma Emerg Surg 2018; 44(1):87–95.

28. Dohan DM, Choukroun J, Diss A, et al. Platelet-Rich Fibrin (PRF): a second-generation platelet concentrate. Part I: technological concepts and evolution.

Oral Surg Oral Med Oral Pathol Oral Radiol Endod 2006;101(3):e37–44.

29. Choukroun J, Diss A, Simonpieri A, et al. Platelet-rich fibrin (PRF): a second-generation platelet concentrate. Part V: histologic evaluation of PRF effect on bone allograft maturation in sinus lift. Oral Surg Oral Med Oral Pathol Oral Radiol Endod 2006;101:29.

30. Litvinov RI, Weisel JW. What is the biological and clinical relevance of fibrin? Semin Thromb Hemost 2016;42(4):333–43.

31. Kumar K, Genmorgan K, Abdul Rahman S, et al. Role of plasma-rich fibrin in oral surgery. J Pharm Bioallied Sci 2016;8. https://doi.org/10.4103/0975-7406.191963. Available at: https://search-proquest-com.libdb.db.uth.tmc.edu/docview/1840794987?accountid=7127.

32. Ghanaati S, Booms P, Anna O, et al. Advanced platelet-rich fibrin: a new concept for cell-based tissue engineering by means of inflammatory cells. J Oral Implantol 2014;40(6):679–89.

33. Dragonas P, Katsaros T, Avila-Ortiz G, et al. Effects of leukocyte–platelet-rich fibrin (L-PRF) in different intraoral bone grafting procedures: a systematic review. Int J Oral Maxillofac Surg 2018. https://doi.org/10.1016/j.ijom.2018.06.003.

34. Alzahrani AA, Murriky A, Shafik S. Influence of platelet rich fibrin on post-extraction socket healing: a clinical and radiographic study. Saudi Dent J 2017;29(4):149–55.

35. Femminella B, Iaconi MC, Di Tullio M, et al. Clinical comparison of platelet-rich fibrin and a gelatin sponge in the management of palatal wounds after epithelialized free gingival graft harvest: a randomized clinical trial. J Periodontol 2016;87(2): 103–13.

36. Bahammam MA. Effect of platelet-rich fibrin palatal bandage on pain scores and wound healing after free gingival graft: a randomized controlled clinical trial. Clin Oral Investig 2018;22(9):3179–88.

37. Miron RJ, Fujioka-Kobayashi M, Bishara M, et al. Platelet-rich fibrin and soft tissue wound healing: a systematic review. Tissue Eng B Rev 2017;23(1): 83–99.

38. Öncü Elif, Alaaddinoğlu E. The effect of platelet-rich fibrin on implant stability. Int J Oral Maxillofac Implants 2015;30(3):578–82.

39. Kim HS, Park JC, Yun PY, et al. Evaluation of bone healing using RhBMP-2 soaked hydroxyapatite in ridge augmentation: a prospective observational study. Maxillofac Plast Reconstr Surg 2017;39(1). https://doi.org/10.1186/s40902-017-0138-9.

40. Spagnoli D, Choi C. Extraction socket grafting and buccal wall regeneration with recombinant human bone morphogenetic protein-2 and acellular collagen sponge. Atlas Oral Maxillofac Surg Clin North Am 2013;21(2):175–83.

41. Chen Di, Zhao M, Mundy GR. Bone morphogenetic proteins. Growth Factors 2004;22(4):233–41.

42. McKay WF, Peckham SM, Badura JM. A comprehensive clinical review of recombinant human bone morphogenetic protein-2 (INFUSE® Bone Graft). Int Orthop 2007;31(6):729–34.

43. Fiorellini JP, Howard Howell T, Cochran D, et al. Randomized study evaluating recombinant human bone morphogenetic protein-2 for extraction socket augmentation. J Periodontol 2005;76(4):605–13.

44. Herford AS. The use of recombinant human bone morphogenetic protein-2 (RhBMP-2) in maxillofacial trauma. Chin J Traumatol 2017;20(1):1–3.

45. Freitas RM, Spin-Neto R, Marcantonio Junior E, et al. Alveolar ridge and maxillary sinus augmentation using RhBMP-2: a systematic review. Clin Implant Dent Relat Res 2015;17(S1):e192–201.

46. Francis CS, Mobin SS, Lypka MA, et al. RhBMP-2 with a demineralized bone matrix scaffold versus autologous iliac crest bone graft for alveolar cleft reconstruction. Plast Reconstr Surg 2013;131(5):1107–15.

47. Medtronic package insert no. M704819B001 (2007) INFUSE® bone graft for Certain oral maxillofacial and dental regenerative uses.

48. Herford AS, Boyne PJ, Rawson R, et al. Bone morphogenetic protein-induced repair of the premaxillary cleft. J Oral Maxillofac Surg 2007;65(11):2136–41.

49. Valdes M, Thakur N, Namdari S, et al. Recombinant bone morphogenic protein-2 in orthopaedic surgery: a review. Arch Orthop Trauma Surg 2009;129(12):1651–7.

50. Holton J, Imam M, Ward J, et al. The basic science of bone marrow aspirate concentrate in chondral injuries. Orthop Rev (Pavia) 2016;8(3):6659. https://doi.org/10.4081/or.2016.6659.

51. Abukawa H, Shin M, Williams WB, et al. Reconstruction of mandibular defects with autologous tissue-engineered bone. J Oral Maxillofac Surg 2004;62(5):601–6.

52. Cassano JM, Kennedy JG, Ross KA, et al. Bone marrow concentrate and platelet-rich plasma differ in cell distribution and interleukin 1 receptor antagonist protein concentration. Knee Surg Sports Traumatol Arthrosc 2016;26(1):333–42.

53. Gimbel M, Ashley RK, Sisodia M, et al. Repair of alveolar cleft defects: reduced morbidity with bone marrow stem cells in a resorbable matrix. J Craniofac Surg 2007;18(4):895–901.

54. Chahla J, Mannava S, Cinque ME, et al. Bone marrow aspirate concentrate harvesting and processing technique. Arthrosc Tech 2017;6:e441–5.

55. Dawson JI, Smith JO, Aarvold A, et al. Enhancing the osteogenic efficacy of human bone marrow aspirate: concentrating osteoprogenitors using wave-assisted filtration. Cytotherapy 2013;15(2):242–52.

56. Warnke PH. Repair of a human face by allotransplantation. Lancet 2006;368(9531):181–3.

57. Konopnicki S, Troulis MJ. Mandibular tissue engineering: past, present, future. J Oral Maxillofac Surg 2015;73(12):136–46.

58. Moghadam HG, Urist MR, Sandor GK, et al. Successful mandibular reconstruction using a BMP bioimplant. J Craniofac Surg 2001;12:119.

59. Warnke PH, Springer ING, Wiltfang J, et al. Growth and transplantation of a custom vascularised bone graft in a man. Lancet 2004;364:766.

60. Kim YH, Furuya H, Tabata Y. Enhancement of bone regeneration by dual release of a macrophage recruitment agent and platelet-rich plasma from gelatin hydrogels. Biomaterials 2014;35:214–24. with permission from Elsevier.

61. Masoudi E, Ribas J, Kaushik G, et al. Platelet-rich blood derivatives for stem cell-based tissue engineering and regeneration. Curr Stem Cell Rep 2016;2(1):33–42.

62. Johnson J, Jundt J, Hanna I, et al. Resection of an ameloblastoma in a pediatric patient and immediate reconstruction using a combination of tissue engineering and costochondral rib graft. J Am Dent Assoc 2017;148(1):40–3.

63. Melville JC, Tursun R, Green JM, et al. Reconstruction of a post-traumatic maxillary ridge using a radial forearm free flap and immediate tissue engineering (bone morphogenetic protein, bone marrow aspirate concentrate, and cortical-cancellous bone): case report. J Oral Maxillofac Surg 2017;75(2). https://doi.org/10.1016/j.joms.2016.11.001.

64. Kim B, Zaid W, Park E, et al. Hybrid mandibular reconstruction technique: preliminary case series of prosthetically-driven vascularized fibula free flap combined with tissue engineering and virtual surgical planning. J Oral Maxillofac Surg 2014;72(9). https://doi.org/10.1016/j.joms.2014.06.013.

65. Asa'ad F, Pagni G, Pilipchuk SP, et al. 3D-printed scaffolds and biomaterials: review of alveolar bone augmentation and periodontal regeneration applications. Int J Dent 2016. https://doi.org/10.1155/2016/1239842.

66. 3D Polymer Scaffolds for Tissue Engineering | Nanomedicine. Available at: https://www.futuremedicine.com/doi/abs/10.2217/17435889.1.3.281. Accessed January 10, 2019.

67. Ceccarelli G, Presta R, Benedetti L, et al. Emerging perspectives in scaffold for tissue engineering in oral surgery. Stem Cells Int 2017. https://doi.org/10.1155/2017/4585401.

68. Fahimipour F, Rasoulianboroujeni M, Dashtimoghadam E, et al. 3D printed TCP-based scaffold incorporating VEGF-Loaded PLGA microspheres for craniofacial tissue engineering. Dent Mater 2017;33(11):1205–16.

69. Cui H, Zhu W, Nowicki M, et al. Hierarchical fabrication of engineered vascularized bone biphasic constructs via dual 3D bioprinting: integrating regional bioactive factors into architectural design. Adv Healthc Mater 2016;5(17):2174–81.

70. Kwee BJ, Mooney DJ. Biomaterials for skeletal muscle tissue engineering. Curr Opin Biotechnol 2017; 47:16–22.

71. Passipieri JA, Christ GJ. The potential of combination therapeutics for more complete repair of volumetric muscle loss injuries: the role of exogenous growth factors and/or progenitor cells in implantable skeletal muscle tissue engineering technologies. Cells Tissues Organs 2016;202(3–4):202–13.

72. Liu J, Saul D, Oliver Böker K, et al. Current methods for skeletal muscle tissue repair and regeneration. Biomed Res Int 2018. https://doi.org/10.1155/2018/1984879.

73. Murphy MK, MacBarb RF, Wong ME, et al. Temporomandibular joint disorders: a review of etiology, clinical management, and tissue engineering strategies. Int J Oral Maxillofac Implants 2013;28(6):e393–414.

The Use of Patient-Specific Implants in Oral and Maxillofacial Surgery

Michael F. Huang, DDS, MD[a,b],*, David Alfi, DDS, MD[a,b], Jonathan Alfi, MA[c], Andrew T. Huang, MD[d]

KEYWORDS

- Patient-specific implants • 3D printed plates
- Custom temporomandibular joint total joint replacement • Maxillofacial reconstruction
- Orthognathic surgery • Computer-aided design • Computer-aided manufacture

KEY POINTS

- Patient-specific cutting guides and patient-specific implants are becoming increasingly common in oral and maxillofacial surgery.
- Custom temporomandibular joint (TMJ) total joint prosthesis allows for individualized reconstruction of the TMJ.
- Computer-aided design and computer-aided manufacturing technology allows for the fabrication of patient-specific cutting guides and patient-specific reconstruction plates used for accurate and efficient reconstruction of complex maxillofacial defects with or without vascularized bone flaps.
- Improved accuracy of patient-specific implants allows for their application in orthognathic surgery, although their use in mandibular surgery, specifically the bilateral sagittal split osteotomy, has yet to be proven.

INTRODUCTION

Personalized medicine is a term that has gained momentum in the twenty-first century. The National Cancer Institute defines it as "a form of medicine that uses information about a person's gene, proteins, and environment to prevent, diagnose, and treat disease."[1] It refers to a shift away from the "one-size-fits-all" approach designed for the average patient toward treatments tailored for the individual. Given the complexity of the facial skeleton and the development of computer-aided design and computer-aided manufacturing (CAD/CAM) technology, several recent developments have allowed the application of personalized medicine to oral and maxillofacial surgery in order to improve outcomes. The decreasing cost of this technology has also made it more affordable and accessible to patients. Patient-specific implants are currently used in multiple areas of oral and maxillofacial surgery, including temporomandibular joint (TMJ) total joint replacement, reconstruction of the maxillofacial skeleton, and orthognathic surgery.

Disclosure Statement: The authors have nothing to disclose.
[a] Department of Oral and Maxillofacial Surgery, Houston Methodist Hospital, 6560 Fannin Street, Suite 1280, Houston, TX 77030, USA; [b] Weill Cornell Medical College, New York, NY, USA; [c] Surgical Planning Laboratory, Department of Oral and Maxillofacial Surgery, Houston Methodist Research Institute, 6560 Fannin Street, Suite 1280, Houston, TX 77030, USA; [d] Otolaryngology – Head & Neck Surgery, Baylor College of Medicine, 1977 Butler boulevard, Suite E5.200, Houston, TX 77030, USA
* Corresponding author. Department of Oral and Maxillofacial Surgery, Houston Methodist Hospital, 6560 Fannin Street, Suite 1280, Houston, TX 77030, USA
E-mail address: mfhuang@houstonmethodist.org

Oral Maxillofacial Surg Clin N Am 31 (2019) 593–600
https://doi.org/10.1016/j.coms.2019.07.010

CONTENT

Temporomandibular Joint Total Joint Replacement

Alloplastic replacement of the entire TMJ complex, including fossa and the condyle-ramus unit, for the treatment of severe end-stage TMJ disease or pathologic condition has been described as early as 1970. Several different alloplastic materials have been used for these devices, including cast Vitallium with a polymethyl methacrylate head,[2] Proplast-Teflon-coated Vitallium,[3] and Dacron/Proplast-Teflon/ultra-high-molecular-weight polyethylene.[4] Patient-specific implants using CAD/CAM technology for TMJ replacement was introduced in 1993.[5] Since then, several studies have validated the long-term stability and success rate of these devices,[6–8] with the longest follow-up being 20 years.[9]

Currently, the only Food and Drug Administration–approved custom-made total joint prosthesis in the United States is one made by TMJ Concepts (Ventura, CA, USA). The workflow begins with a computed tomographic (CT) scan following their protocol in order to fabricate a stereolithic skull model from which the mandibular resection and fossa preparation can be performed. A minimum gap of 13 mm should be present from the skull base to the mandible after the resection. The postresection stereolithic skull model is then shipped to TMJ Concepts for implant design and fabrication that is specific to the patient's anatomic morphology, surgical defect, and jaw relationship. TMJ Concepts' fossa component is made from unalloyed titanium mesh bonded to an articulating surface made of ultra-high-molecular-weight polyethylene. Their mandibular component is composed of a condylar head made from cobalt-chromium-molybdenum alloy and a mandibular body made from titanium-aluminum-vanadium extralow interstitial alloy.[10] A third-party virtual surgical planning software (ie, 3D Systems, Materialise, or Individual Patient Solutions) can be used to fabricate intraoperative cutting guides in order to replicate the planned resection and joint reconstruction.

A study involving 45 patients published in 2003 demonstrated better outcomes with custom TMJ prostheses fabricated by TMJ Concepts (formerly Techmedica Inc) compared with stock prostheses made by TMJ Inc.[11] A recent meta-analysis did not reveal any relevant differences between stock and patient-specific prostheses with respect to increased maximum incisal opening and decreased pain.[12] Although TMJ total joint replacement can be reliably performed using a stock prosthesis in a more timely fashion because of the longer processing time required for skull models and custom implants, there are many advantages to using custom-made prostheses, including reconstruction of complex defects of the skull base and mandible (**Fig. 1**) as well as greater ability to alter the position of the mandible in relation to the skull base as seen in concomitant TMJ reconstruction and orthognathic surgery.[13]

Reconstruction of the Maxillofacial Skeleton

There are many challenges unique to bony reconstruction of the maxillofacial skeleton, including anatomic diversity, complex movement of the mandible, saliva contamination, and dental rehabilitation. Internal fixation in maxillofacial surgery gained popularity after the introduction of antibiotics in the 1940s.[14] Christiansen[15] is

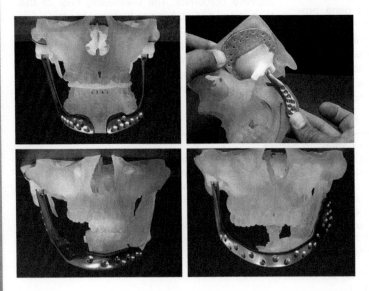

Fig. 1. Reconstruction of complex surgical defects involving the TMJ, skull base, and hemimandible using custom TMJ prostheses. (*Courtesy of* TMJ Concepts, Inc., Ventura, CA.)

credited with introducing bone plates to maxillo-facial surgery in 1945, but most surgeons at that time used plates and screws designed for ortho-pedics (ie, metacarpal plates). Luhr[16] was the first to study rigid internal fixation for maxillofa-cial surgery and introduced compression plates as well as self-threading screws to the specialty in the 1960s. Before the development of custom implants, mandibular reconstruction was carried out using rigid fixation plates and locking screws designed to fit the "average" mandible, usually at the inferior border away from relevant anatomic structures, such as inferior alveolar neurovascu-lar bundle and teeth. The titanium reconstruction plates were flat and required bending intraoper-atively while the patient remained under general anesthesia, after adequate exposure is achieved and sometimes after resection had taken place. Some prefabricated plates had a built-in angle to simulate the in-plane bend at the angle of the mandible. Despite this, shaping a mandibular reconstruction plate to fit a particular patient's surgical defect was time consuming and weak-ened the integrity of the plate.

A major advancement to patient-specific im-plants was the rapid prototyping of stereolithic models to scale, first described in oral and maxil-lofacial surgery by Brix and Lambrecht[17,18] in 1987. The printed models can be used to manu-ally bend reconstruction plates fitted for a partic-ular defect before the day of surgery, a concept commonly known as "prebending." This tech-nique allowed for the accurate adaptation of the reconstruction plate to the patient's anatomy without the patient being under anesthesia with an open wound. As the prices of desktop 3-dimensional (3D) printers and resins decreased over time, it became feasible and practical for in-dividual institutions to fabricate stereolithic models on their own using in-house CAD soft-ware (ie, Anatomic Aligner). Improved accuracy of prebent plates compared with the conven-tional method of intraoperative bending for mandibular reconstruction was demonstrated in a study of 42 patients in 2015.[19] The drawback of plate weakness that occurs with bending how-ever still remains, although at lesser values because of more direct and improved application.

The first case report of a patient-specific plate used in mandibular reconstruction was in 2012 by Ciocca and colleagues,[20] whereby a titanium alloy plate was manufactured by direct metal laser sintering using a CAD/CAM protocol to reconstruct a mandibular defect from oral can-cer. Similar to the fabrication of a custom TMJ prosthesis, this protocol begins with sending the DICOM data of the preoperative CT scan to the medical engineers at a third-party virtual surgical planning company (ie. 3D Systems [Lit-tleton, CO, USA], Materialise [Leuven, Belgium], Individual Patient Solutions [Breisgau, Ger-many]). The recommended slice thickness of the CT scan is less than 1.0 mm in order to have adequate surface detail on which accurate surgical guides and implants can be manufac-tured. A Web meeting then takes place between the surgeon and the engineer to plan the resec-tion, design the surgical guides, and design the reconstruction plate. The surgical guide serves as a cutting guide for the resection as well as a drill guide for the screws used to secure the reconstruction plate. After the Web meeting, a report is e-mailed to the surgeon for final design approval before manufacturing. The cutting guides, reconstruction plate, an optional steriliz-able stereolithic model, and a detailed report of the surgical plan are sent to the surgeon before surgery (Fig. 2). A multicenter study of 30 pa-tients in 2015 validated this protocol for recon-struction of mandibular defects using patient-specific surgical guides and patient-specific implants.[21]

Mascha and colleagues[22] demonstrated the accuracy of mandibular reconstruction using patient-specific mandibular reconstruction plates milled from titanium blocks, with slightly better results in sole alloplastic reconstruction cases compared with cases whereby osseous flap reconstruction was performed. When used in conjunction with composite flap reconstruction (ie, fibula, iliac crest, and scapula) of complex mandibular defects, patient-specific cutting and drilling guides that correspond to patient-specific reconstruction plate allow for accurate 3D orientation of the bony flap segments. The accuracy of flap reconstruction compared with the virtual plan in 6 patients was evaluated by Schepers and colleagues,[23] who found a mean deviation of 3.0 mm (standard deviation 1.8 mm) and a mean angulation of 4.2° (standard deviation 3.2°). One factor that accounts for the decreased accuracy of fibula reconstruction compared with virtual plan is the fit of fibula cutting guides over an intact periosteum, which is arbitrarily determined to be 0.4 mm during CAD/CAM fabrication of the surgical guide. Although this study had a small sample size, it likely reflects greater accuracy and precision compared with conventional techniques of free-hand reconstruction and intraoperative bending, not to mention decreased surgical times. The same study also evaluated the accuracy of endosseous implants placed at the time of

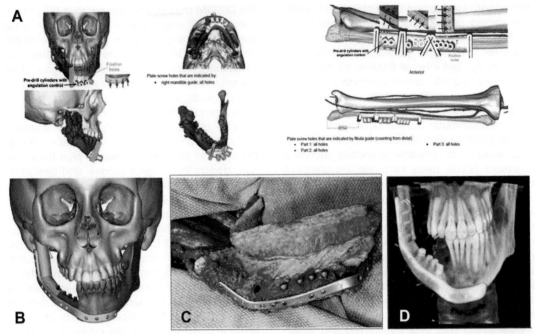

Fig. 2. Reconstruction of a mandibular ramus-condyle unit using vascularized fibula flap. (*A*) Custom cutting guides for the resection and flap harvest. (*B*) Virtual plan of the flap reconstruction with planned dental implants. (*C*) Assembled fibula flap using patient-specific reconstruction plate with dental implants inserted using the custom drill guides built into the fibula cutting guide. (*D*) Postoperative CT scan demonstrating the final reconstruction.

primary reconstruction using patient-specific drill guides and found deviation of 2.2 mm (standard deviation 1.1 mm) and 10.7° angular deviation (standard deviation 7.6°). This deviation again likely reflects the decreased accuracy of adaptation of the fibula drilling guide on the fibula on account of the periosteum, which is needed to maintain vascularity. Two recent studies compared fibula reconstruction of mandibular defects using patient-specific implants with the conventional method of prebending. There was a greater degree of deviation from the virtual plan in the conventional method, but this difference was not statistically significant.[24,25]

Reconstruction of the maxilla and orbitozygomatic regions is equally challenging given the complex 3D anatomy as well as its multiple functions, including separation of the oral and nasal cavities, and support for dentition. Melville and colleagues[26] published a case report of fibula reconstruction of a maxillary defect (Brown classification IId) using patient-specific guides and patient-specific implants. The overall workflow is very similar to mandibular reconstruction using a vascularized flap. The patient-specific reconstruction plate allowed for accurate orientation of the fibula segments in order to reconstruct the alveolar portion of the surgical defect. The customized

plate allowed for the placement of screws in areas of native bone with predicable thickness (ie, buttresses).

Orthognathic Surgery

Orthognathic surgery has been revolutionized by advances in 3D imaging and CAD/CAM technology. Traditional orthognathic surgery involves presurgical planning using 2-dimensional cephalometric analysis, facebow transfer, plaster models, and an Erickson model table. The model surgery is then transferred to the operating room using occlusal wafers, and surgery is carried out using miniplates that are adapted intraoperatively. Thanks to the work by Gateno, Xia, and other pioneers, this method has been replaced with digital planning using 3D data, but the surgical plan is still transferred to the patient using occlusal wafers printed based on "intermediate" and "final" occlusions. Although 3D surgical planning provides significant foresight into issues that can be encountered intraoperatively (ie, proximal and distal segment collision during sagittal split osteotomy and bony interferences during Le Fort I impaction), the surgery does not exactly replicate the surgical plan because the osteotomies are still made freehand. In

2013, Li and colleagues[27] published a series of 6 patients who underwent Le Fort I osteotomy using 3D printed cutting and repositioning guides whereby the final maxillary position was determined using bone-borne guides, independent of occlusion or the position of the mandible. This technique eliminated the potential errors caused by autorotation of the mandible, but fixation of the final maxillary position was achieved using the conventional technique of intraoperative plate bending, which is technique sensitive and has the ability to introduce errors.

The first case report of patient-specific implants used in orthognathic surgery in the English literature was published by Philippe[28] in 2013. In this report, they described a patient who underwent segmental Le Fort I osteotomy using bone-borne cutting guides that also served as a drill guide for final fixation. After downfracture and mobilization of the Le Fort I segments, fixation was performed using 3 laser-sintered custom implants secured using the predrilled holes. Minimal discrepancy in plate position was seen between the virtual surgical plan and postoperative result. The exclusive use of bone-borne patient-specific guides and patient-specific implants avoided the need for occlusal wafers. Two larger studies published in 2015 and 2016 described the use of patient-specific cutting guides and patient-specific implants for Le Fort I osteotomy in 10 and 32 patients, respectively.[29,30] Precise fit of the 3D printed plates was seen in most cases. Unacceptable fit of the custom implants was seen in only 1 case in Suojanen and colleagues[30'] study, and the remainder of the surgery was carried out using a CAD/CAM occlusal wafer and traditional plate bending.

In 2017, Heufelder and colleagues[31] published a series of 22 patients who underwent bimaxillary orthognathic surgery. In this series, all patients underwent maxilla surgery first using patient-specific bone-borne guides and patient-specific implants manufactured by selective laser melting. After repositioning of the maxilla using the waferless technique, mandibular surgery was carried out in conventional fashion using CAD/CAM occlusal wafers in the final position and intraoperative bending of fixation plates. When postoperative results were compared with the presurgical plan, they found median deviations of 0.3 mm in the left-right dimension plane, 0.33 mm in the vertical dimension, and 0.7 mm in the anterior-posterior dimension.

There are several advantages to maxillary positioning using patient-specific cutting guides and patient-specific implants: (1) accurate 3D positioning of the maxilla independent of occlusion or the position of the mandible; (2) elimination of intraoperative plate bending, which is time consuming, weakens the integrity of the bone plates and can introduce errors; (3) elimination of intermaxillary fixation, which is also time consuming and puts personnel at risk for penetrating injuries; and (4) precise placement of screw using patient-specific drill guides designed to for placement in thick bone and to avoid key areas such as dental roots. Disadvantages of patient-specific implants used in Le Fort I osteotomy for orthognathic surgery include (1) increased cost, some of which may be offset by decreased time in the operating room; (2) increased processing time for fabrication of the patient-specific guides and implants; (3) inability to change the plan intraoperatively in cases where the virtual plan is not accurately translated to the patient; (4) risk of screw placement in thin maxillary bone without the ability to alter screw placement; and (5) unpredictability of maxillary transverse stability in cases of segmental maxillary surgery.

Suojanen and colleagues[32] evaluated the use of patient-specific osteotomy and drill guides and milled patient-specific implants in 30 patients who underwent mandibular advancement with bilateral sagittal split osteotomy. They found accurate fit of the implants in 11 patients, acceptable fit after modifications in 17 patients, and unacceptable fit in 2 patients. This inaccuracy is likely due to the unpredictability in seating the proximal segment and imprecise preoperative virtual prediction of the sagittal split. The investigators thus recommended that patient-specific implants should not be used without occlusal wafers. Around the same time, a group from China published a series of 10 patients who underwent splintless bimaxillary surgery using patient-specific implants for the maxilla and mandible.[33] They noted small differences in position and orientation between the planned and postoperative outcomes, but stated "all the patients achieved good final occlusion without postoperative elastic traction."

In the series published by Heufelder and colleagues,[31] all patients underwent bimaxillary surgery with the maxilla-first approach using patient-specific implants followed by mandibular surgery using CAD/CAM occlusal wafers and internal fixation via the conventional approach. This sequence allowed for accurate 3D positioning of the maxillomandibular complex with establishment of appropriate final occlusion, which may not be achieved with fully guided orthognathic surgery exclusively using bone-borne guides and patient-specific implants

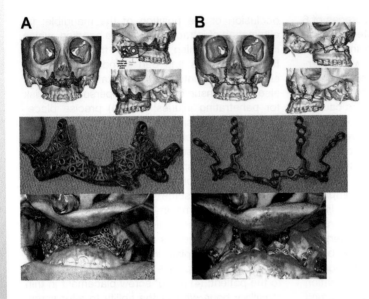

Fig. 3. Orthognathic surgery using patient-specific cutting guides (*A*) and patient-specific implants (*B*).

(**Fig. 3**). Because establishment of normal occlusion is a major goal of orthognathic surgery, this seems to be a prudent approach of incorporating patient-specific implants into orthognathic surgery.

Future Direction

Autogenous bone grafting remains the gold standard for reconstruction of the maxillofacial skeleton because the biomechanical properties best match that of the missing tissue it is meant to replace. In certain areas of reconstruction, patient-specific titanium alloy implants are used for accurate positioning and fixation of autogenous bone grafts (ie, vascularized fibula and non-vascularized iliac crest). In other areas, such as TMJ reconstruction and orbital fracture repair,

sole reconstruction using alloplastic materials has become more popular because of the better customization of the implants and avoidance of donor site morbidity with low rate of complications. Ideally, reconstruction using an autogenous material identical to the surgical defect in size and shape would be best for restoration of form and function. Advances in tissue engineering using scaffolds and stem cells will soon allow for reconstruction of bony defects using autogenous bone without the need for significant donor site morbidity.

Patient-specific custom implants made with autogenous, adipose-derived, stem cells (ASCs) in custom bioreactors have already proven efficacy and superiority to traditional implants in large animal studies. Bhumiratana and colleagues[34] demonstrated that anatomically correct bone

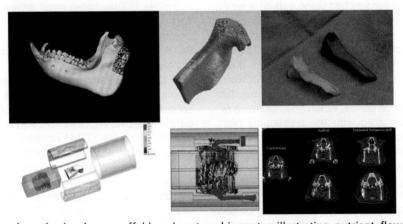

Fig. 4. Custom shape bovine bone scaffold and custom bioreactor illustrating nutrient flow for stem cell manipulation.

grafts from ASCs were grown and implanted in Yucatan mini-pigs to reconstruct the ramus-condyle unit (**Fig. 4**). The custom stem cell grafts were tested against both no graft and scaffold only and were found to have superior characteristics in terms of strength, volume, and shape. The stem cell grafts were also found to benefit from antiresorptive properties.

The need for reconstruction alternatives with synthetic availability that allows for single-staged procedures and avoids donor site morbidity is paramount to the evolution of patient-specific implants. Fortunately, advances in technology and biomaterials provide us with a real opportunity to introduce regenerative products that can be printed in the desired shape, size, form, and architecture. Tools that are readily printable and have the advantage of sterility, antimicrobial properties, and regenerative capability provide for very exciting possibilities. Years of development have brought us to this point, where we are ready to test and develop this technology.

SUMMARY

Patient-specific implants are oral and maxillofacial surgery's answer to personalized medicine. Although this technology has been in use for many years in some areas such as TMJ total joint replacement, it is relatively new in other areas, such as reconstruction and orthognathic surgery. Advances in CAD/CAM technology with decreasing costs will continue to allow this field to evolve in order to improve accuracy, efficiency, and overall outcome.

REFERENCES

1. National Cancer Institute. NCI dictionary of cancer terms. Available at: https://www.cancer.gov/publications/dictionaries/cancer-terms. Accessed February 1, 2019.

2. Christensen RW. Arthroplastic implantation of the TMJ. In: Cranin A, editor. Oral Implantology. Springfield: Charles C Thomas; 1970. p. 284–98.

3. Hinds EC, Homsy CA, Kent JN. Use of a biocompatible interface for binding tissues and prosthesis in temporomandibular joint surgery. Oral Surg Oral Med Oral Pathol 1974;38:512–9.

4. Kent JN, Block MS, Halpern J, et al. Long-term results on VK partial and total temporomandibular joint systems. J Long Term Eff Med Implants 1993;3(1):29–40.

5. Henry CH, Wolford LM. Treatment outcomes for temporomandibular joint reconstruction after Proplast-Teflon implant failure. J Oral Maxillofac Surg 1993;51:352–8.

6. Mercuri LG, Wolford LM, Sanders B, et al. Custom CAD/CAM total temporomandibular joint reconstruction system: preliminary multicenter report. J Oral Maxillofac Surg 1995;53(2):106–15.

7. Mercuri LG, Giobbie-Hurder A. Long-term outcomes after total alloplastic temporomandibular joint reconstruction following exposure to failed materials. J Oral Maxillofac Surg 2004;62(9):1088–96.

8. Mercuri LG, Edibam NR, Giobbie-Hurder A. Fourteen-year follow-up of a patient-fitted total temporomandibular joint reconstruction system. J Oral Maxillofac Surg 2007;65(6):1140–8.

9. Wolford LM, Mercuri LG, Schneiderman ED, et al. Twenty-year follow-up study on a patient-fitted temporomandibular joint prosthesis: the Techmedica/TMJ Concepts device. J Oral Maxillofac Surg 2015;73(5):952–60.

10. TMJ Concepts. Material Description. Available at: https://tmjconcepts.com/product-information/material-description/. Accessed February 1, 2019.

11. Wolford LM, Dingwerth DJ, Talwar RM, et al. Comparison of 2 temporomandibular joint total joint prosthesis systems. J Oral Maxillofac Surg 2003;61:685–90.

12. Zou L, He D, Ellis E. A comparison of clinical follow-up of differential total temporomandibular joint replacement prostheses: a systematic review and meta-analysis. J Oral Maxillofac Surg 2018;76:294–303.

13. Movahed R, Teschke M, Wolford LM. Protocol for concomitant temporomandibular joint custom-fitted total joint reconstruction and orthognathic surgery utilizing computer-assisted surgical simulation. J Oral Maxillofac Surg 2013;71:2123–9.

14. Ellis E. Rigid skeletal fixation of fractures. J Oral Maxillofac Surg 1993;51:163–73.

15. Christiansen GW. Open operation and tantalum plate insertion for fracture of the mandible. J Oral Surg 1945;3:194.

16. Luhr HG. Zur stabilen osteosynthese bie unterkieferfrakturen. Dtsch Zahnarztl Z 1968;23:754.

17. Brix F, Lambrecht JT. Preparation of individual skull models based on computed tomographic information. Fortschr Kiefer Gesichtschir 1987;32:74–7.

18. Lambrecht JT, Brix F. Individual skull model fabrication for craniofacial surgery. Cleft Palate J 1990;27(4):382–5.

19. Wilde F, Winter K, Kletsch K, et al. Mandible reconstruction using patient-specific pre-bent reconstruction plates: comparison of standard and transfer key methods. Int J Comput Assist Radiol Surg 2015;10:129–40.

20. Ciocca L, Mazzoni S, Fantini M, et al. CAD/CAM guided secondary mandibular reconstruction of a continuity defect after ablative cancer surgery. J Craniomaxillofac Surg 2012;40:e511–5.

21. Wilde F, Hanken H, Probst F, et al. Multicenter study on the use of patient-specific CAD/CAM reconstruction plates for mandibular reconstruction. Int J Comput Assist Radiol Surg 2015;10:2035–51.

22. Mascha F, Winter K, Pietzka S, et al. Accuracy of computer-assisted mandibular reconstructions using patient-specific implants in combination with CAD/CAM fabricated transfer keys. J Craniomaxillofac Surg 2017;45:1884–97.

23. Schepers RH, Raghoebar GM, Vissink A, et al. Accuracy of fibula reconstruction using patient-specific CAD/CAM reconstruction plates and dental implants: a new modality for functional reconstruction of mandibular defects. J Craniomaxillofac Surg 2015;43:649–57.

24. Mazzoni S, Marchetti C, Sgarzani R, et al. Prosthetically guided maxillofacial surgery: evaluation of the accuracy of a surgical guide and custom-made bone plate in oncology patients after mandibular reconstruction. Plast Reconstr Surg 2013; 131(6):1376–85.

25. Ciocca L, Marchetti C, Mazzoni S, et al. Accuracy of fibular sectioning and insertion into a rapid-prototyped bone plate, for mandibular reconstruction using CAD-CAM technology. J Craniomaxillofac Surg 2015;43:28–33.

26. Melville JC, Manis CS, Shum JW, et al. Single-unit 3D-printed titanium reconstruction plate for maxillary reconstruction: the evolution of surgical reconstruction for maxillary defects–a case report and review of current techniques. J Oral Maxillofac Surg 2018. https://doi.org/10.1016/j.joms.2018.11.030.

27. Li B, Zhang L, Sun H, et al. A novel method of computer aided orthognathic surgery using individual CAD/CAM templates: a combination of osteotomy and repositioning guides. Br J Oral Maxillofac Surg 2013;51:e239–44.

28. Philippe B. Custom-made prefabricated titanium miniplates in LeFort I osteotomies: principles, procedure and clinical insights. Int J Oral Maxillofac Surg 2013;42:1001–6.

29. Mazzoni S, Bianchi A, Schiariti G, et al. Computer-aided design and computer-aided manufacturing cutting guides and customized titanium plates are useful in upper maxilla waferless repositioning. J Oral Maxillofac Surg 2015;73:701–7.

30. Suojanen J, Leikola J, Stoor P. The use of patient-specific implants in orthognathic surgery: a series of 32 maxillary osteotomy patients. J Craniomaxillofac Surg 2016;44:1913–6.

31. Heufelder M, Wilde F, Pietzka S, et al. Clinical accuracy of waferless maxillary positioning using customized surgical guides and patient specific osteosynthesis in bimaxillary orthognathic surgery. J Craniomaxillofac Surg 2017;45:1578–85.

32. Suojanen J, Leikola J, Stoor P. The use of patient-specific implants in orthognathic surgery: a series of 30 mandible sagittal split osteotomy patients. J Craniomaxillofac Surg 2017;45:990–4.

33. Li B, Shen S, Jiang W, et al. A new approach of splint-less orthognathic surgery using a personalized orthognathic surgical guide system: a preliminary study. Int J Oral Maxillofac Surg 2017;46: 1298–305.

34. Bhumiratana S, Bernhard JC, Alfi DM, et al. Tissue-engineered autologous grafts for facial bone reconstruction. Sci Transl Med 2016;8(343):ra83.

Practice Management in Oral and Maxillofacial Surgery

James Baker, DDS[a], Austin Leavitt, MS, CFP®[b], Jonathon S. Jundt, DDS, MD[c],*

KEYWORDS

- Practice management • Marketing • Electronic medical records • Revenue cycle management
- Coding • Benefits

KEY POINTS

- This article reviews the rise and role of dental service organizations, management service organizations, private equity, and trends in practice transitions.
- This article reviews marketing oral and maxillofacial surgery services, including search engine optimization and reputation management.
- This article reviews practice revenue cycle management, including changes in the insurance industry, coding, billing, and the role of the electronic health records and real-time insurance authorization.
- This article reviews essential terms and past and current trends in the management of oral and maxillofacial surgery practices to discuss the current state of practice and to develop predictions about the future of the specialty.

INTRODUCTION

Managing an oral and maxillofacial surgery (OMS) practice has undergone dramatic changes. Electronic health records, privacy laws, revenue cycle management, online marketing, and the rise of dental service organizations (DSOs) present increased daily complexity for oral and maxillofacial surgeons in private practice, hospital-based employees, and academic surgeons. This article is structured to discuss the role of DSOs, private equity in OMS, online practice marketing, accounting and tax considerations, and modern essentials of practice management.

DENTAL SERVICE ORGANIZATIONS

DSOs, also referred to as dental support organizations, represent the fastest growing segment in oral health care.[1] Strategies for network growth vary from a de novo practice development model to acquisition-based growth or a combination thereof. Services provided often include revenue cycle management, information technology, marketing, human resources, and financial reporting. Services are provided on an a la carte or comprehensive basis. DSO funding may be through private equity or venture capital or evolve from a group of one large or multiple existing practices. The objectives of a DSO are to standardize the provision of health care to patients through reducing nonclinical burdens on the providers. Student loan burdens on new providers reduce the likelihood of purchasing a practice or starting a de novo solo practice on the completion of training. A general trend in health care toward increased consolidation and decreased private

Disclosure: The authors have nothing to disclose.

[a] OMS Partners, 5599 San Felipe Street, Suite 900-B, Houston, TX 77056, USA; [b] The Financial Advisory Group, 5599 San Felipe, Suite 900, Houston, TX 77056, USA; [c] Department of Oral and Maxillofacial Surgery, The University of Texas Health Science Center at Houston, 7500 Cambridge Street, Suite 6100, Houston, TX 77054, USA
* Corresponding author.
E-mail address: jonathon.jundt@uth.tmc.edu

Oral Maxillofacial Surg Clin N Am 31 (2019) 601–609
https://doi.org/10.1016/j.coms.2019.07.004
1042-3699/19/© 2019 Elsevier Inc. All rights reserved.

ownership continues.[1] This trend is partly fueled by the challenges of maximizing insurance reimbursement, variations in scope of practice, increasing population, limited negotiating power of individual practices, complexity of staff management and benefits, and generational psychology. DSOs provide the organizational capacity to facilitate increased practice revenue through economies of scale and represent a growing and substantial component of delivering OMS services in the future.

The authors' experience has determined a cost of approximately 9.5% of practice revenue to deliver services in this type model. Services provided under this structure vary by the DSO but should include revenue cycle management, credentialing, annual fee analysis, human resources, payroll, payment of practice bills, employee and doctor benefit management, information technology support, accounting—monthly profit and loss or financials through corporate tax returns, regulatory compliance, and cash flow management. Services provided and fees charged vary by the DSO involved.

New versions of DSOs are now entering the market and provide services in addition to the aforementioned list, which now include direct-to-consumer marketing, group purchasing organizations, quality-of-life products, regional surgery centers, call coverage, insurance negotiation, and the facilitation of practice transitions. Fees currently marketed are in the 15–18% of total practice revenue. One theory supporting this growth is that the excess revenue to the DSO creates a large enough profit that can be sold at a multiple large enough to provide more to the OMS selling their practice in the marketplace as well as a return to the DSO. Several examples of this DSO model are funded by outside investors, such as private equity. Some models involve a sale of the practice assets that may involve a funding mechanism through a hedge fund or other entity. Other similar models exist that do not require a practice asset sale but do involve a larger fee, with the same goal of gaining a return on the excess revenue greater than the OMS has relinquished for the service.

Complexities facing private practice oral and maxillofacial surgeons and new graduates alike are resulting in a shift toward the DSO model. The type of practice model that will be commonplace in the future is to be determined and historically has been subject to political and regulatory changes.

PRIVATE EQUITY

Private equity investors seek to generate a return on high-growth investments for pension funds, high net worth individuals, institutional investors, and sovereign wealth funds. Although private equity and venture capital are sometimes discussed in the same context, they are very different funding mechanisms. Private equity rarely invests in start-ups, focusing on mature companies, whereas venture capital commonly invests in start-ups. Private equity typically acquires the majority of a company, whereas venture capital typically owns a small percentage of a company. Dermatology and ophthalmology underwent extensive private equity acquisitions in the late 1990s and early 2000s. The model for investment was an upfront payment to the practice as a multiple of collections, followed by a reinvestment in the group by acquired practice owners and a contract to continue to work for the new group at a reduced income to improve earnings before interest, depreciation, taxes, and amortization (EBIDTA). Once the practice financials demonstrated growth and profitability, a second sale is undertaken to a third party at a larger multiple than the initial buyout, thus financially rewarding the private equity investors and those practitioners who reinvested and participated in the second sale.

MARKETING

Google was founded 20 years ago. Since that time, OMS practice marketing changed dramatically. Health care consumers began the transition from trusting their provider recommendation to shopping for health care. A simple search query now yields millions of results in milliseconds, processing 40,000 searches per second, 3.5 billion per day, and 1.2 trillion searches per year. Patients discover practices in a geographic designation based on the parameters set by their ad campaign. This trend does not show signs of slowing, with older computer-illiterate generations leaving the marketplace and younger computer-savvy generations fully embracing technology. Search engine optimization marries the information displayed by a practice Web site with those search queries initiated by the individual. Furthermore, targeted advertisements may appear as banners on social media because of recent queries, GPS tracking, or passive smartphone listening capabilities.[2,3] Optimization requires active participation in Web site design and formatting as well as communication and marketing through major search engines. Reputation management has also evolved as dissatisfied patients are able to use the Internet as a platform to discuss their particular complaints in an open forum, often resulting in a star rating for the practitioner. Several companies now provide reputation management and offer strategies to avoid or eliminate negative reviews. One mechanism for reputation management involves contacting patients via text or email after services are rendered, requesting a review. The screen is often a simple thumbs-up or thumbs-down icon or a recommended or not recommended icon. Patients select the icon that best fits their experience. If patients selects a negative review, the service redirects their review to an internal quality-control response that requests additional information about their experience, forwarding the results to the practitioner. Should patients report a positive review, they are redirected to a public external domain with a request to elaborate on their positive experience. This mechanism improves practice reviews by redirecting those with negative experiences to a site isolated from the public domain.

Search engine optimization works through a combination of outbidding competitors within a marketplace, insight into the timing and nature of client searches, demographics, keywords, type of device accessed, and Web site design. Cost per click, impressions, and click-through rates are tabulated to assess advertising effectiveness (**Fig. 1**). The click-through rate measures how often people click an ad on viewing. Impressions are recorded each time the advertisement is presented online to an individual browsing the Internet. Cost per click is the amount paid to the advertising agency after an individual clicks the link to access the advertisement. This amount

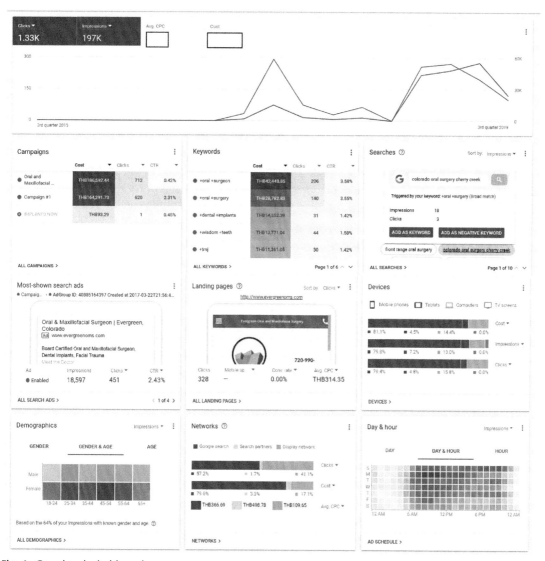

Fig. 1. Google ads dashboard.

is stipulated in advance with limits. Competitors are limited through intelligent algorithms that detect repeated clicking to exhaust a budget with the intent of removing the ad. In the continually expanding era of "Internet of things," patients likely will own their chart information on their personal devices and schedule appointments, follow-ups, procedures, medications, and complications on their personal devices.

PRACTICE FINANCE

Countless developments in research through regenerative medicine, 3-D printing, real-time robotic surgical adjuncts, and advanced imaging portend a bright future replete with enhanced surgical ability and improved patient outcomes. Societal needs for specialist services constitute a pinnacle in the hierarchy of patient care, which remains relevant. Providing those services to the public requires functional and effective business models to implement care efficiently, safely, and in a manner that sustains the practitioners and attracts new talent to the field. Without an understanding of accounting, taxes, profit and loss, and revenue cycle management, the financial health of a practice could be in jeopardy.

ACCOUNTING AND TAX

Recent tax changes arose from the Tax Cuts and Jobs Act of 2017.[4] Pertinent aspects of this legislation to the practitioner include

- Increased standard deduction
- Elimination of personal exemption
- Reducing alternative minimum tax and eliminating it for corporations

- Increased state tax exemption for individuals and couples
- General decreases in ordinary income tax
- Decrease in C-corporation tax from 35% to 21%.
- Introduction of a 20% pass-through deduction for qualifying businesses
- Limiting the state tax deduction against federal tax to $10,000

One change that is frequently asked by practitioners, or S-corporations, that own member interests in a partnership is in regard to the 20% pass-through deduction or section 199A. Despite initial enthusiasm over potential benefits this could provide to surgeons, the final bill primarily benefitted manufacturers and other businesses not classified as "service" companies.

If taxable income married filing jointly (MFJ) is below $415,000, a phased-out deduction may be qualified for. For a majority of practitioners, however, the 20% pass-through deduction yields little to no additional tax benefit (**Fig. 2**). Regardless of the potential for decreased tax savings according to the aforementioned chart (**Fig. 2**), there may be benefits to maintaining an entity tax status as an S corporation. These benefits may include

1. Avoidance of double taxation associated with C corporations
2. The tax reductions from proactive tax planning and classification of form W-2 and schedule K-1 income from the entity. **Table 1** compares types of income and the applicable tax.

Income classified as form W-2 is subject to federal income tax, state income tax, social security tax, Medicare tax, and Medicare surtax. Schedule

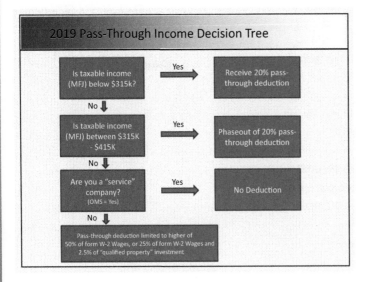

Fig. 2. Pass-through income decision tree.

Table 1 Tax comparison		
Tax	Form W-2	Schedule K-1
Federal income tax	Taxable at ordinary income tax rate	Taxable at ordinary income tax rate
State income tax	Taxable at ordinary income tax rate	Taxable at ordinary income tax rate
Social Security tax	6.2%–12.4% taxable up to $132,900 (2019)	
Medicare tax	1.45%–2.9% taxable	
Medicare surtax	0.9% above $250,000 (MFJ, 2019)	

K-1 income is subject only to federal income tax and state tax where applicable. The temptation is to classify little to nothing as form W-2 income and classify everything as schedule K-1. This generally is not recommended. Although the Internal Revenue Service has not traditionally offered exact guidance on this issue, the idea is that surgeon owners should pay themselves a "reasonable salary" classified as form W-2 income, which fulfills the intended tax revenue goals of the treasury. Also, form W-2 income is considered earned income whereas schedule K-1 income is not. Earned income is necessary for the deferment and utilization of multiple and complex retirement vehicles. Without earned income, surgeon cannot defer. Because tax scenarios can vary widely, counsel of a certified public accontant (CPA) or trusted advisors should be sought on this issue.

TRANSITIONS

Surgeons at each phase of their career enjoy multiple opportunities and challenges. Whether retiring from practice, graduating from residency, or transitioning from associateship to ownership, it is important to meticulously analyze the opportunity prior to entering into a contract. **Fig. 3** compares 3 practice settings available to new graduates.

Separate from determining what kind of work a surgeon wants to pursue, there is also the question of association with third-party firms for fulfilling business processes. As evidenced in other specialties, an ever-increasing compliance burden and decreasing insurance reimbursement environment is leading many surgeons to engage in larger practice partnerships, DSO groups, or management service organizations (MSO). Each of these come with risks and benefits that should be contemplated prior to entering into a new engagement. **Fig. 4** compares traditional partnerships with the DSO and MSO models of practice.

For an acquisition and depending on the entity type acquired, there may be more than 1 option for completing the transaction. Although beyond the scope of this article, certain transactions may yield higher post-tax benefit through capital gains treatment as opposed to ordinary income. Any contemplated transaction should also be reviewed

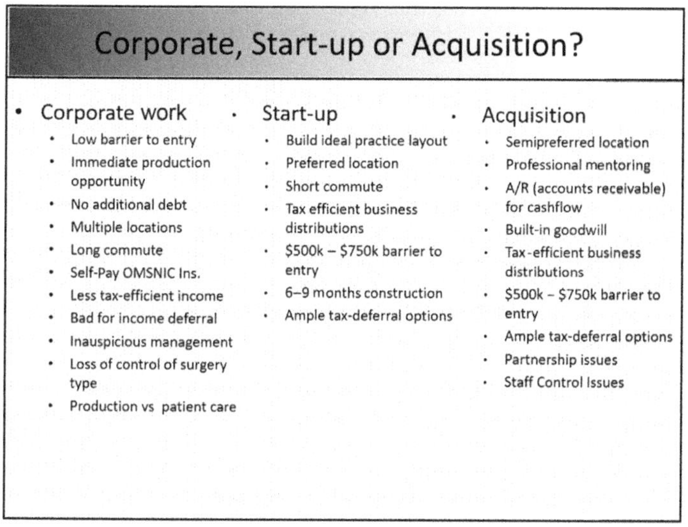

Fig. 3. Transition comparison.

Corporate, Start-up or Acquisition?

- Corporate work
  - Low barrier to entry
  - Immediate production opportunity
  - No additional debt
  - Multiple locations
  - Long commute
  - Self-Pay OMSNIC Ins.
  - Less tax-efficient income
  - Bad for income deferral
  - Inauspicious management
  - Loss of control of surgery type
  - Production vs patient care

- Start-up
  - Build ideal practice layout
  - Preferred location
  - Short commute
  - Tax efficient business distributions
  - $500k – $750k barrier to entry
  - 6–9 months construction
  - Ample tax-deferral options

- Acquisition
  - Semipreferred location
  - Professional mentoring
  - A/R (accounts receivable) for cashflow
  - Built-in goodwill
  - Tax-efficient business distributions
  - $500k – $750k barrier to entry
  - Ample tax-deferral options
  - Partnership issues
  - Staff Control Issues

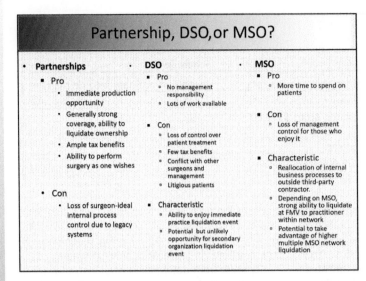

Fig. 4. Partnership, DSO, and MSO comparison. FMV, Fair Market Value.

thoroughly by legal counsel, CPAs, certified financial planners, and trusted advisors with knowledge on the subject.

MODERN ESSENTIALS OF PRIVATE PRACTICE

Following the 3 As of new practice development was a private practice adage for many years. Availability, affability, and ability were the key elements of a successful medical practice. Accounting and advertising are becoming increasingly important in the modern practice and may expand the 3 As to 5 As. This list contains some basic terms essential to understanding the financial health of a practice (**Table 2**). These terms provide information on practice metrics like profitability and earnings for a practitioner. These include

- Base salary
- Taxes
- Travel and lodging
- Continuing education
- Auto
- 401(k)/profit sharing
- Defined benefit or cash balance plan
- Insurance
- Marketing

A plan should be in place to legally minimize the tax burden by maximizing all the other items listed.

Direct operating costs deserve analysis. Approximately 80% of direct operating costs are fixed costs, such as rent, that do not vary based on how many patients are seen or procedures performed. Only approximately 20% of these costs vary based on the volume of patients seen or procedures performed. A simple way to illustrate this helps understand its importance.

In an average OMS practice, collecting $100,000 per month with a 50% overhead, $40,000 is spent because the practice exists. Another $10,000 is spent on available direct cost, leaving approximately $50,000 for the OMS to utilize. Indirect costs amount to another $5000 to $10,000 per month, reducing available compensation to approximately $40,000 to $45,000. This example illustrates the power of marginal revenue. Once the fixed costs are covered, additional

Table 2 Financial terms	
Term	**Definition**
Gross revenue	Total receipts
Net revenue	Total receipts minus patient and insurance refunds
Adjustments	The difference in the fee schedule and what the third-party payer contracted with allow or pays for a code
Production	Total charges based on fees
Collections	Total amount of money received
Direct operating cost	Actual expenses to have a practice open
Indirect operating cost	Interest, depreciation, taxes, amortization
EBIDTA	Earnings before interest, depreciation, taxes, and amortization
Accounts receivable	Fees billed but not yet collected

Table 3 Marginal revenue comparison		
Revenue	$100,000	$120,000
Direct operating	$50,000	$52,400
Indirect operating	$10,000	$10,000
Available	$40,000	$57,600

revenue has only a 20% overhead. If an additional $20,000 per month is collected, approximately $16,000 goes to OMS compensation, with only $4000 of additional overhead. **Table 3** demonstrates the relationship and power of marginal revenue.

In a group of more than 50 oral and maxillofacial surgeons whose practice data are available to the authors, the average net collection per OMS is approximately $1,360,000. After direct and indirect expenses, the available money to use for the OMS is approximately 45%, or $612,000.

Retirement plans, including 401(k) and pension funding, although included in overhead, do provide additional benefit to the business owner and should be considered when calculating an owner's total financial benefit. Derived from the sample group of practices, the average percentage of operating cost allocations as a percentage of collections is illustrated in the **Fig. 5**.

Profit and loss statements, balance sheet analysis, and entity tax returns comprise a standard practice financial analysis. A profit and loss statement is what most practitioners utilize to demonstrate overall profitability of the practice. After the available operating income (net from direct operating cost) has been determined, a few noncash adjustments for depreciation and amortization. With the remainder amount, form W-2 or schedule K-1 income can be classified with the help of a CPA.

REVENUE CYCLE MANAGEMENT

Revenue cycle management is the process of billing and collecting revenue. It has expanded to include credentialing. Credentialing has become a complex undertaking. This is how a doctor becomes a provider for third-party payers, obtains hospital staff privileges, obtains all licenses and permits at the state and federal levels, and joins various state and national organizations.

The revenue cycle begins with the patient encounter. The encounter is recorded with a diagnosis code, and any interventions performed, including an examination, imaging, or surgical intervention, require procedure code. Only 1 fee goes with each code with few exceptions. These exceptions are documented with a modifier, indicating a more simple or more complex procedure, and the fee can be higher or lower. A flow diagram may be beneficial to visualize the process, allowing for objective evaluation of the billing lifecycle, and provides an avenue to alter processes to maximize outcomes for the practice. A basic diagram (**Fig. 6**) should be followed to insure a proper workflow from consult to compensation.[5] Correct coding takes place both after the initial consult and is again verified after the treatment is completed.

The codes are used to generate a bill to a patient who pays a portion and a third-party payer pays a portion. If the OMS is a contracted provider with a third-party payer, it is likely that the accepted fee will be lower than the standard fees. This difference is called an adjustment or write-off. Inherent in this process is an occasional overpayment by a patient or a third-party payer. This amount must then be refunded to the patient or insurance plan. At the end of each month, there is a cycle of production, adjustments, collections, and refunds, which results in net collections. Net

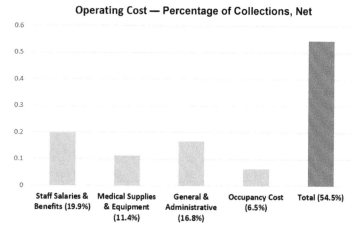

Operating Cost — Percentage of Collections, Net

Fig. 5. Operating cost.

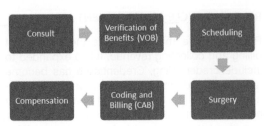

Fig. 6. Insurance cycle.

1. Precontract models, now called out of network
2. In-network provider
3. Corporate employee
4. Hospital or large medical group provider/employee

There also are at least 3 locations as potential practice patterns:

1. Office only
2. Hospital and office
3. Hospital only

collections then pay direct and indirect operating expenses.

A practice generally is owed money by patients and insurance plans. The amounts are known as accounts receivable and a practice management system produces a monthly production/collection report that includes an aged accounts receivable report to those over 120 days. Amounts aged beyond 120 days are unlikely to be collected in a significant amount. **Table 4** lists examples of aged accounts receivable reports for a practice performing dentoalveolar only and 1 performing a mix of dentoalveolar and medically coded procedures. The percentage in the table represents an ideal or expected distribution of accounts receivable by age. The larger percent greater than 120 days with medical procedures is due to the large number of uninsured patients requiring treatment of facial trauma and infections through emergency treatment in this example.

Revenue to the OMS consist of accounts paid by patients in the office, known as time of service, and revenue paid from accounts receivable. An average practice receives 35% from time of service and 65% from accounts receivable. These percentages vary based on the variety of procedures performed and the amount of managed care plans accepted.

In the past, medical or dental services were provided and the patients paid the bills. As insurance matured and expanded, patients continued to pay the bills and received reimbursement by their insurance plan. These are precontract delivery models. Below is a list of common practice models:

Due to the large variety of procedures under the scope of OMS, all models have the ability to provide a profitable and gratifying career. In general, the greater the prevalence of dental procedures and codes, the simpler and faster the revenue cycle. As procedures commonly performed in a hospital or an outpatient surgical center increase, the revenue cycle slows. This is not a negative. With either situation, once the cycle has been running for 6 months or more, the revenue flow stabilizes, with the practice in solid financial shape. Revenue cycle management affords insight into the cyclical timing of cash flows. **Fig. 7** lists is the average cyclical cash flow timing for single provider with single-location engagements.

Because of the delay in the timing of insurance receivables, the cyclical nature of procedures performed follows a similar pattern to average net collections illustrated in **Fig. 7**. The cyclical delay will be impacted by the percentage of insurance procedures performed (as opposed to the percentage of self-pay patients), the insurance companies a practice is contracted with, and the billing & coding processes & procedures utilized. Summer is often the most productive period for an OMS and the winter season less productive. As a practical business application, high collections in August may be used to complete any unfunded 401(k) or pension liabilities accrued from prior tax year because these need to be fully funded by September after the given tax year.

Now emerging is the OMS version of a concierge medical practice. The OMS is contracted to a hospital or large medical entity with the majority of the compensation delivered as a salary. At

Table 4					
Aged accounts receivable expected values					
	Current	**31–60 d**	**61–90 d**	**91–120 d**	**Greater than 120 d**
Dentoalveolar	58%	18%	6%	4%	14%
Dentoalveolar/medical	60%	10%	5%	5%	20%

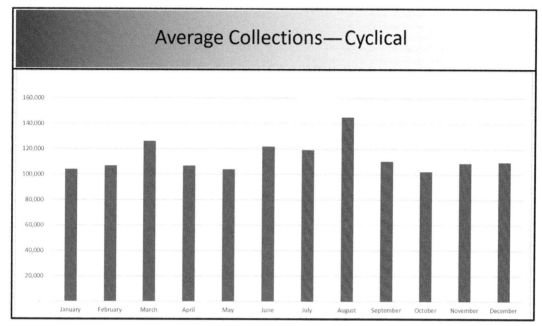

Fig. 7. Average cyclical collections, single practice.

this time there remains additional compensation per procedure performed, but most of the revenue comes as salary. The authors have observed this to be a growing niche, and it may develop into a major part of the intersection of the OMS specialty with the medical model.

SUMMARY

The practice of OMS continues to evolve. Private practice delivery of care is intrinsically dependent on sound financial processes and a robust understanding of the revenue cycle, marketing, purchasing, staff management, insurance nuances, and credentialing. Consolidation in medicine and dentistry by large corporations continues to gain market share at a time when student loan debts have reached historically high levels, leading to an increasing percentage of graduates seeking employment supplemented by independent contractor work at the offices of nonspecialists. If OMS as a specialty mirrors those of other surgical specialties, the increased complexity of delivering health care could result in a sustained decrease in private practice ownership.

REFERENCES

1. Vujicic M. Practice ownership is declining. J Am Dent Assoc 2017;148(9):690–2.
2. Available at: https://www.vice.com/en_uk/article/wjbzzy/your-phone-is-listening-and-its-not-paranoia. Accessed August 5, 2019.
3. Available at: https://www.cbsnews.com/news/phone-listening-facebook-google-ads/. Accessed August 5, 2019.
4. Available at: https://www.irs.gov/newsroom/tax-cuts-and-jobs-act-provision-11011-section-199a-qualified-business-income-deduction-faqs. Accessed August 5, 2019.
5. Jundt J. Dictations and coding in oral and maxillofacial surgery. Houston (TX): MD2B; 2018.

Fig. 7. Average clinical collections, single practice.

Advances in Anesthesia Monitoring

Yi Deng, MD[a],*, Jovany Cruz Navarro, MD[b,c], Sandeep Markan, MD[a]

KEYWORDS

- Anesthesia monitoring • Perioperative monitoring • Neurologic monitoring
- Cardiovascular monitoring

KEY POINTS

- There have been many advances in perioperative anesthetic monitoring, specifically in the fields of neurologic and cardiovascular monitoring.
- Neurologic monitoring is necessary to prevent nerve injury, ensure adequate depth of anesthesia, and optimize cerebral oxygenation.
- Minimally invasive cardiovascular monitors use dynamic measures of fluid responsiveness to better assess and manage the patient's volume status.

INTRODUCTION

Patient monitoring during the administration of anesthesia is essential for safety and a core tenet of anesthesiology. The American Society of Anesthesiology established guidelines and promotes minimum practice standards of monitoring cardiopulmonary function and perfusion. These include heart rate and rhythm, blood pressure (BP), temperature, oxygenation, and ventilation. Adjunctive monitoring techniques and advances in neurologic, neuromuscular, and cardiovascular monitoring further enhance the practitioner's ability to provide safe and effective anesthesia. Topics selected for inclusion in this article focus on those monitoring elements most germane to oral maxillofacial surgery (OMS).

NEUROLOGIC MONITORING

Neural function is essential for cognition and to the hallmark of human existence. A permanent loss of neural function because of anesthesia complications during surgery is a major loss to the individual. Advances during the last three decades have led to improvements in clinical neuromonitoring technology. The goal of neuromonitoring is to assess and preserve the functional integrity of the brain, brainstem, spinal cord, and/or peripheral nerves during surgery. If mechanical or physiologic injury to these structures is suspected, neuromonitors can alert the anesthesiologist and surgeon to allow modification of treatment strategies. In OMS procedures, intricate work is often done near major nerves and vascular structures, which may require special anesthetic techniques. Neuromonitoring techniques include cerebral oxygen monitoring, processed electroencephalography (pEEG), electromyography (EMG), evoked potentials (EP), somatosensory EP (SSEP), brainstem auditory EP, and visual EP. This section explores the details of advances in neuromonitoring.

Disclosure Statement: The authors have nothing to disclose.
[a] Department of Anesthesiology and Critical Care Medicine, Baylor College of Medicine, 1 Baylor Plaza, MSC 120, Houston, TX 77030, USA; [b] Department of Anesthesiology, Baylor College of Medicine, 1 Baylor Plaza, MSC 120, Houston, TX 77030, USA; [c] Department of Neurosurgery, Baylor College of Medicine, Houston, TX, USA
* Corresponding author.
E-mail address: yd1@bcm.edu
twitter: @chrisdengMD (Y.D.)

Cerebral Oxygenation Monitoring

Cerebral oxygenation (O_2) monitoring should be instituted during general anesthesia whenever there is concern of intraoperative cerebral ischemia, as in patients with known severe carotid stenosis, extremes in head positioning, and/or existing intracranial abnormalities combined with large expected blood loss. There are many modalities for directly monitoring cerebral O_2 (ie, mixed jugular venous saturation, partial brain tissue O_2), but these are invasive in nature and require a neurosurgeon. One new technology marketed over the last decade is near-infrared spectroscopy (NIRS), which places two small pads on the patient's forehead that continuously and noninvasively monitor regional cerebral O_2 saturation.[1]

NIRS devices measure the transmission of near-infrared light and its differential absorption by chromophores (usually oxyhemoglobin and deoxyhemoglobin) across brain tissues. This absorption difference correlates to the degree of tissue O_2 saturation. Unlike conventional pulse oximetry, NIRS interrogates arterial, venous, and capillary blood in totality as a weighted value that does not require pulsatile flow to function. Currently it is used to guide brain-protective strategies during cardiac surgery,[2] carotid endarterectomy,[3] endovascular therapy for acute ischemic stroke,[4] and traumatic brain injury monitoring.[5] The normal range of regional cerebral O_2 saturation is between 55% and 75%, although substantial intraindividual and interindividual variability exists. A significant drop can suggest ongoing cerebral ischemia, which may necessitate maneuvers, such as raising O_2 delivery (eg, augmenting cardiac output [CO], transfusing red blood cells) or lowering O_2 extraction (eg, treating fever and infection, reducing work of breathing).

Evidence supporting the routine use of NIRS is currently limited. One must be wary that its value can be influenced by many factors, such BP, hemoglobin concentration, and cerebral blood volume. In addition, there is potential for "signal contamination" by extracranial tissue (ie, scalp hematoma, scalp itself, or thick cranium).[1,6] Furthermore, the sensitivity of global cerebral ischemia detection is likely limited by the small sampling area in the frontal cortex.[1]

Electroencephalography

Standard electroencephalography interpretation is cumbersome, requires professional interpretation, and is not routinely used in the operating room except in certain neurosurgical procedures. However, in the last 20 years there has been an increase in pEEG monitoring, used anywhere from complex cardiac surgery to outpatient hernia repair. Today, they are commonly used during general anesthesia cases to monitor the depth of anesthesia. The most widely available device is the bispectral index monitor, which processes frontal electroencephalography signals to derive a score between 0 and 100. Values greater than 90 suggest wakefulness, whereas less than 60 suggest general anesthesia.[7]

The pEEG monitors have been postulated to ensure adequate depth of anesthesia, decrease the risk of intraoperative awareness, and postoperative cognitive dysfunction. So far, the evidence is equivocal.[8,9] Similar to NIRS, many factors affect pEEG signal and therefore its interpretation. Nevertheless, if inhalational anesthetics are contradicted because of either patient or surgical factors, pEEG monitoring may be helpful to guide the depth of anesthesia using intravenous (IV) anesthetics during surgery.

Electromyography

EMG is used to monitor cranial or peripheral nerves at risk of surgical injury, and is commonly deployed during OMS procedures. EMG can identify direct mechanical trauma to the nerve, which is seen as high-frequency neurotonic discharges (**Fig. 1**).[10] In addition, it is used to identify nerves that are otherwise difficult to visualize. When an innervated muscle is triggered by stimulation, a compound muscle action potential is recorded.[11]

When monitoring EMG during spinal surgery, an increase in compound muscle action potential latency can indicate nerve injury, and the surgeon

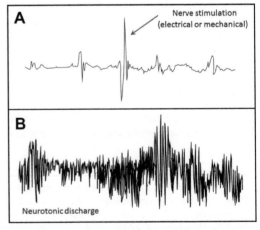

Fig. 1. (*A*) Electromyography recording showing a large isolated response from electric or mechanical stimulation. (*B*) Nerve stretch or mechanical trauma can cause continuous, high-frequency recordings known as neurotonic discharges, suggestive of nerve injury.

may need to act to mitigate further damage (ie, halt electrocautery activity in the proximity, decrease screw or plate tension).

Similarly, cranial nerve (CN) monitoring is a form of EMG and shares the same principles, although only CNs with motor component can be monitored (CN III, IV, V, VI, VII, IX, X, XI, and XII).[12]

Evoked Potentials

EP monitoring is used to assess the integrity of a neural pathway. It typically involves stimulating peripheral sites of the body and recording responses centrally (opposite for motor EP [MEP]). The amplitude and latency of such recorded waveforms are analyzed to provide functional neurologic assessment. A 50% decrease in waveform amplitude and/or a 10% increase in latency may indicate nerve dysfunction and/or injury, and necessitate modification in surgical strategy, patient positioning, and anesthetic management.[13]

SSEP is the most commonly used EP monitoring modality. An electrical stimulus is applied to a peripheral nerve in the upper or lower extremity and measured with scalp electrodes (**Fig. 2**). It is particularly useful during spine surgery because it monitors the integrity of the dorsal root ganglia and the dorsal columns.[14] MEPs, however, use transcranial electrical stimulation and monitor the corticospinal tract, nerve roots, and peripheral nerves.[15] MEPs are more effective than SSEPs in detecting motor neuron injury because changes there precede that of SSEPs. Other commonly used modalities include brainstem auditory EPs for posterior fossa surgeries and visual EPs for procedures near the occipital lobe.

Most currently available anesthetics alter neural function by producing dose-dependent depression in synaptic activity. As such, the anesthetic effects vary with the location of the synapses. In general, inhalational agents have greater effects on EPs than do IV agents. Choice and dosage of anesthetics should be tailored to the desired EP monitoring technique. In addition, physiologic factors (ie, anemia, hypothermia, hypotension, hypoxia) and patient positioning (ie, severe neck flexion) can all affect EP assessment.

NEUROMUSCULAR MONITORING

Neuromuscular blocking agents (NMBAs) or muscle relaxants were introduced in 1942 by Griffith and Johnson and are commonly used in OMS. In recent years, increased recognition of postoperative residual paralysis and its associated dangers has led to greater emphasis on improved monitoring and routine reversal to decrease its incidence. Newly published guidelines[16] recommend the use of quantitative, objective measurements instead of traditional subjective measurements. Subjective monitoring refers to visual or tactile evaluation of the train-of-four (TOF) count or degree of TOF fade in response to peripheral neurostimulation (**Fig. 3**). It is the defacto standard used today. Recent evidence indicates that a TOF ratio greater than or equal to 0.9 (as opposed to the traditionally taught 0.7) is necessary for safe extubation and decreased postoperative residual paralysis.[17,18] However, physicians tend to overestimate TOF ratio when using subjective evaluation[19] and are unable to accurately detect fade when TOF ratio is greater than 0.4.[20]

Quantitative monitors include acceleromyography, which can accurately detect fade, TOF count, and TOF ratio. It is a finger-sized device placed on the thumb and measures its acceleration in response to ulnar nerve stimulation. Some caveats to use include mandatory calibration and unimpeded movement of the thumb during surgery. Kinemyography is another quantitative monitor

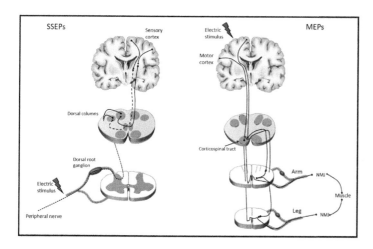

Fig. 2. Typical neural pathways assessed with SSEP and MEP monitoring. SSEPs are produced by stimulation of a peripheral nerve and measured centrally. MEPs are produced by stimulation of the motor cortex and measured peripherally. NMJ, Neuromuscular junction.

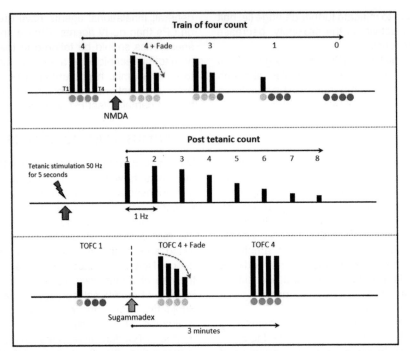

Fig. 3. Neuromuscular blockade monitoring with TOF count and TOF fade. In profound block when TOF count is 0, one can provide tetanic stimulation for 5 seconds and count the number of posttetanic twitches to estimate degree of blockade. Sugammadex can reverse deep blockade to a TOF count of 4 within 3 minutes, which is not possible with neostigmine.

that measures the electrical signal generated from the distortion of a mechanosensor, which is placed between the base of the thumb and index finger. Its results are not interchangeable with other quantitative modalities, and the technology has similar limitations as the acceleromyography.[21] Finally, previously described EMG can also objectively monitor the neuromuscular function recovery, although its use is much more cumbersome.

Although there has not been a novel NMBA approved clinically in some time, sugammadex has been introduced recently as a reversal agent. Sugammadex is a γ-cyclodextrin, which selectively binds free plasma steroidal NMBA molecules, rendering them unavailable for redistribution in the neuromuscular junction. Affinity is greatest for rocuronium, followed by vecuronium, pancuronium, and pipecuronium.[22] It offers rapid and complete reversal (<3 minutes) in usual clinical scenarios and can even reverse profound rocuronium-induced blockade otherwise not possible with neostigmine (see **Fig. 3**).[23] Currently it is not recommended in dialysis patients, and side effects although rare can include interference with oral contraceptive pills, anaphylaxis, cardiac arrhythmias,[24] coronary vasospasm,[25] and mild prolongation of coagulation values.[26] Nevertheless, its availability has profound effects on

anesthetic management, such as preferred choice between succinylcholine and rocuronium for rapid-sequence induction when there are concerns for difficult airway management.

CARDIOVASCULAR MONITORING

Until the last decade, cardiovascular monitoring in anesthesia and surgery had essentially remained unchanged for many years. Conventional measurement of heart rate and rhythm as depicted by five-lead electrocardiogram and BP using automated cuffs and/or intra-arterial catheter are well-accepted methods and have long been incorporated into American Society of Anesthesiology practice guidelines. For higher acuity patients, central venous access is required to either obtain central venous pressure or allow for the insertion of a pulmonary artery catheter (PAC). More recently, however, there has been a substantial increase in new technology centered around cardiac monitoring, which has greatly expanded the clinician's armamentarium and led to better understanding of patient management perioperatively. We briefly review these new methods categorized into minimally invasive and noninvasive groups, followed by a discussion on new markers of fluid responsiveness.

Minimally Invasive Cardiovascular Monitoring

CO obtained from a PAC using thermodilution calculations has been considered gold standard for the last 40 years.[27] However, because of concerns about its invasive nature, perceived deficits in efficacy, and applicability, PAC use has generally been declining since the 1990s.[28,29] In the mid-2000s, several devices have emerged including PiCCO (Pulsion Medical System, Feldkirchen, Germany), LiDCO (LiDCO, London, UK), and FloTrac/Vigileo (Edwards Lifesciences Irvine, CA, USA), which use the pulse contour analysis technology and made it feasible to derive stroke volume (SV) and CO monitoring without the risks of PAC insertion.[30,31]

Pulse contour analysis uses waveforms captured by the arterial line transducer and feeds them into a proprietary algorithm unique to each device. The output variables include SV, SV variation, CO, and systemic vascular resistance. The first device to market using this technology was the PiCCO system in 2000. PiCCO system still required a central line and arterial line to function, but was generally well validated across diverse patient populations and useful in certain groups, such as children where PAC is too large to be inserted.[32–34] Another advantage of the PiCCO system is that intrathoracic blood volume and extravascular lung water can be calculated, which is useful in managing patients with severe lung disease. Pulse contour analysis continuously provides real-time CO monitoring, although external recalibration is required periodically using traditional thermodilution methods. Because central venous access is necessary for its function, it has since given way to less invasiveness techniques, such as LiDCO and FloTrac.

LiDCOplus system (LiDCO, London, UK) is another calibrated device similar to PiCCO. However, instead of using cold saline for thermodilution CO calculation, it uses lithium as an indicator.[35] This allows it to function without a central line, because lithium can be injected through a peripheral IV and picked up by a sensor attached to the arterial line. The device is recalibrated every 8 hours (similar to PiCCO). Disadvantages include chronic lithium therapy and nondepolarizing NMBAs invalidate results, and lithium is contraindicated in first trimester pregnancy.[36–38] In general, LiDCO is also well validated in a variety of patient populations, and is precise compared with the other systems described here.[35,39,40]

Finally, one of the newest devices to market is the FloTrac/Vigileo system. It is unique in that it is an uncalibrated system, and calculates CO and SV using pulse contour analysis alone. To do so it factors in patient's age, gender, weight, and height, and inputs these variables along with the

Table 1
Minimally invasive and noninvasive cardiac output monitoring devices

Device Name	Technology Used	Advantage	Disadvantage
Minimally Invasive			
PiCCO	Pulse contour analysis	Continuous CO monitoring, external calibration for precision, well validated	Central access required
LiDCO	Pulse contour analysis	Continuous CO monitoring, external calibration for precision, well validated, no central access	Lithium injection required, contraindicated in pregnancy, can interfere with chronic lithium therapy or NMBA
FloTrac/ Vigileo	Pulse contour analysis	Continuous CO monitoring, easy to use, no calibration required	Least accurate of the 3, inconsistent tracking, prone to drift over time
Noninvasive			
ClearSight	Pulse contour analysis	Finger cuff used without need for intra-arterial access	Not well validated
TEB	Bioimpedance	Continuous CO monitoring, easy to place	Not well validated, changes in thoracic fluid volume can impede with results
TTE	Ultrasound, Doppler	Highly accurate, well validated, easy to establish diagnosis in experienced hands	Operator dependent, requires training, only intermittent measurement

Abbreviations: TEB, thoracic electrical bioimpedance; TTE, transthoracic echocardiography.

patient's hemodynamic profile into its software algorithm against a dataset of internally validated subjects. Because it lacks external calibration, it is prone to drift and has limited accuracy in critically ill patients with wide swings in systemic vascular resistance, severe arrhythmias, aortic regurgitation, and poor arterial waveform.[41] The company has so far released four iterations of its algorithm software and has improved its accuracy in hyperdynamic and vasoplegic patients, but not in cardiac, liver transplantation, or abdominal aortic aneurysm surgeries.[42–45] Despite these concerns, because of its ease of implementation (Flo-Trac adapter can be connected to existing arterial

transducer setup), it has gained extensive popularity across a wide variety of operating room and intensive care unit cases (**Table 1**).

Noninvasive Cardiovascular Monitoring

Two noninvasive CO monitoring techniques developed recently include the ClearSight system (Edwards Lifesciences) and thoracic electrical bioimpedance. ClearSight uses the same pulse contour analysis principle but uses finger cuffs with LED emitters to obtain waveforms instead of intra-arterial catheters. Thoracic electrical bioimpedance places electrodes across the thorax

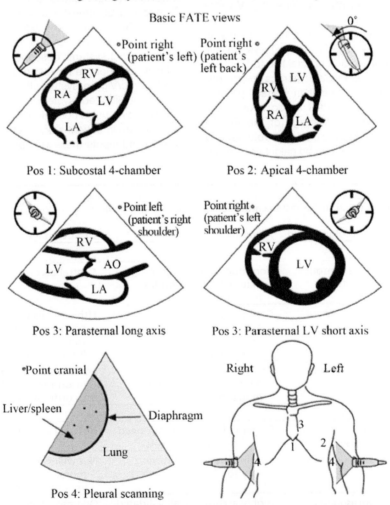

Fig. 4. The basic 4 views of Focus Assessed Transthoracic Echocardiography (FATE) protocol. AO, aorta; LA, left atrium; LV, left ventricle; RA, right atrium; RV, right ventricle. (*From* Oveland N, Bogale N, Waldron B, et al. Focus assessed transthoracic echocardiography (FATE) to diagnose pleural effusions causing haemodynamic compromise. Case Reports in Clin Med. 2013;2(3):190.)

and detects changes in electrical impedance as blood flow in the thoracic aorta varies during cardiac cycle. The limitations of both devices include narrow patient selection, high percent error compared with PACs, and low overall precision.[46–48]

In recent years, point-of-care ultrasound has surged in popularity because of the greater availability and declining cost of portable ultrasound machines. Perioperative transthoracic echocardiography (TTE) brings another dimension to cardiovascular monitoring, enabling a clinician to more accurately assess volume status, cardiac function, and presence of structural heart disease. A complete echocardiographic examination requires significant training and expertise. However, multiple abridged protocols have been developed, such the Focus Assessed Transthoracic Echocardiography and Rapid Assessment by Cardiac Echo, to allow perioperative clinicians rapid evaluation of key identifiers of cardiovascular aberrations.[49,50] In Focus Assessed Transthoracic Echocardiography protocol, for example, only four views are necessary for a complete evaluation (**Fig. 4**). TTE is also superior to catheter-based pressure measurements (eg, PAC) in that cardiac chamber volume can now be directly calculated instead of inferred from pressure-volume curve. Unlike the pulse contour analysis technique, TTE can directly measure SV and CO and is much less prone to biases. Lastly, point-of-care ultrasound can make rapid and accurate diagnosis of other systemic pathologies, such as pneumothorax, consolidations, effusions, and intra-abdominal hemorrhage, thus making it an invaluable tool in the modern perioperative setting.

DYNAMIC MARKERS OF RESUSCITATION

Given the penetration of these cardiovascular monitoring devices, multiple new markers of dynamic volume responsiveness have since come into vogue. It has been recognized that 40% of critically ill and hypotensive patients are actually fluid responsive and can benefit from fluid therapy, whereas excess fluid loading can increase mortality.[51,52] Traditional static measurements of fluid status, such as central venous pressure, have been shown to be extremely poor predictors of volume status and volume responsiveness.[53,54] The most commonly used dynamic markers of fluid resuscitation include pulse pressure variation (PPV), SV variation, and systolic pressure variation, all of which are obtained with the new pulse contour analysis devices.[55] Similarly, TTE can provide clinicians with inferior vena cava

Table 2
Dynamic indices of fluid responsiveness and their accuracy

	Sensitivity (%)	Specificity (%)	AUC
PPV >12%	63	92	0.81
SPV >9%	47	92	0.82
SVV >10%	56	69	0.70
IVCci >15%	31	97	0.62
ΔSV >12%	69	89	0.90

Abbreviations: ΔSV, change in stroke volume after fluid challenge; AUC, area under the receiver operating characteristic curve; IVCci, inferior vena cava collapsibility index; SPV, systolic pressure variation; SVV, stroke volume variation.

collapsibility index, E wave velocity, and aortic velocity time index variations.[56] Each of these markers has independent cutoff values for sensitivity and specificity (**Table 2**). For example, a hypotensive patient with concomitant PPV greater than 12% suggests that the patient can benefit from fluid resuscitation. One must be aware of the pitfalls of each marker in specific clinical scenarios, such as decreased accuracy of PPV in spontaneously breathing patients or those with high intrathoracic or intra-abdominal pressures. Nevertheless, these dynamic markers of fluid resuscitation have proven superiority over static measures, and have shown a high correlation with PAC and TTE.[56] When used with goal-directed fluid therapy, it could potentially reduce the amount of fluid resuscitation, decrease length of stay, postoperative ileus, and prolonged mechanical ventilation, resulting in enhanced recovery after surgery and anesthesia.[55,57]

SUMMARY

In this article, we provide a concise and focused review on the new advances in perioperative neurologic, neuromuscular, and cardiovascular monitoring. It is imperative for surgeons and anesthesiologists to have detailed understanding of the function and limitation of each device to safely guide patients through their surgeries.

REFERENCES

1. Ghosh A, Elwell C, Smith M. Review article: cerebral near-infrared spectroscopy in adults: a work in progress. Anesth Analg 2012;115(6):1373–83.
2. Zheng F, Sheinberg R, Yee M-S, et al. Cerebral near-infrared spectroscopy monitoring and neurologic

outcomes in adult cardiac surgery patients: a systematic review. Anesth Analg 2013;116(3):663–76.

3. Badenes R, García-Pérez ML, Bilotta F. Intraoperative monitoring of cerebral oximetry and depth of anaesthesia during neuroanesthesia procedures. Curr Opin Anaesthesiol 2016;29(5):576–81.

4. Goyal M, Demchuk AM, Menon BK, et al. Randomized assessment of rapid endovascular treatment of ischemic stroke. N Engl J Med 2015;372(11):1019–30.

5. Leal-Noval SR, Cayuela A, Arellano-Orden V, et al. Invasive and noninvasive assessment of cerebral oxygenation in patients with severe traumatic brain injury. Intensive Care Med 2010;36(8):1309–17.

6. Davie SN, Grocott HP. Impact of extracranial contamination on regional cerebral oxygen saturation: a comparison of three cerebral oximetry technologies. Anesthesiology 2012;116(4):834–40.

7. Liu J, Singh H, White PF. Electroencephalographic bispectral index correlates with intraoperative recall and depth of propofol-induced sedation. Anesth Analg 1997;84(1):185–9.

8. Punjasawadwong Y, Phongchiewboon A, Bunchungmongkol N. Bispectral index for improving anaesthetic delivery and postoperative recovery. Cochrane Database Syst Rev 2014;(6):CD003843.

9. Messina AG, Wang M, Ward MJ, et al. Anaesthetic interventions for prevention of awareness during surgery. Cochrane Database Syst Rev 2016;(10):CD007272.

10. Holland NR. Intraoperative electromyography. J Clin Neurophysiol 2002;19(5):444–53.

11. López JR. Neurophysiologic intraoperative monitoring of the oculomotor, trochlear, and abducens nerves. J Clin Neurophysiol 2011;28(6):543–50.

12. Jameson LC, Sloan TB. Monitoring of the brain and spinal cord. Anesthesiol Clin 2006;24(4):777–91.

13. Toleikis JR, American Society of Neurophysiological Monitoring. Intraoperative monitoring using somatosensory evoked potentials. A position statement by the American Society of Neurophysiological Monitoring. J Clin Monit Comput 2005;19(3):241–58.

14. Banoub M, Tetzlaff JE, Schubert A. Pharmacologic and physiologic influences affecting sensory evoked potentials: implications for perioperative monitoring. Anesthesiology 2003;99(3):716–37.

15. Lall RR, Lall RR, Hauptman JS, et al. Intraoperative neurophysiological monitoring in spine surgery: indications, efficacy, and role of the preoperative checklist. Neurosurg Focus 2012;33(5):E10.

16. Checketts MR, Alladi R, Ferguson K, et al. Recommendations for standards of monitoring during anaesthesia and recovery 2015: Association of Anaesthetists of Great Britain and Ireland. Anaesthesia 2016;71(1):85–93.

17. Eikermann M, Blobner M, Groeben H, et al. Postoperative upper airway obstruction after recovery of the train of four ratio of the adductor pollicis muscle from neuromuscular blockade. Anesth Analg 2006;102(3):937–42.

18. Eikermann M, Groeben H, Hüsing J, et al. Accelerometry of adductor pollicis muscle predicts recovery of respiratory function from neuromuscular blockade. Anesthesiology 2003;98(6):1333–7.

19. Brull SJ, Silverman DG. Visual and tactile assessment of neuromuscular fade. Anesth Analg 1993;77(2):352–5.

20. Capron F, Fortier L-P, Racine S, et al. Tactile fade detection with hand or wrist stimulation using train-of-four, double-burst stimulation, 50-hertz tetanus, 100-hertz tetanus, and acceleromyography. Anesth Analg 2006;102(5):1578–84.

21. Stewart PA, Freelander N, Liang S, et al. Comparison of electromyography and kinemyography during recovery from non-depolarising neuromuscular blockade. Anaesth Intensive Care 2014;42(3):378–84.

22. Bom A, Hope F, Rutherford S, et al. Preclinical pharmacology of sugammadex. J Crit Care 2009;24(1):29–35.

23. Sørensen MK, Bretlau C, Gätke MR, et al. Rapid sequence induction and intubation with rocuronium-sugammadex compared with succinylcholine: a randomized trial. Br J Anaesth 2012;108(4):682–9.

24. Bhavani SS. Severe bradycardia and asystole after sugammadex. Br J Anaesth 2018;121(1):95–6.

25. Okuno A, Matsuki Y, Tabata M, et al. A suspected case of coronary vasospasm induced by anaphylactic shock caused by rocuronium-sugammadex complex. J Clin Anesth 2018;48:7.

26. Rahe-Meyer N, Fennema H, Schulman S, et al. Effect of reversal of neuromuscular blockade with sugammadex versus usual care on bleeding risk in a randomized study of surgical patients. Anesthesiology 2014;121(5):969–77.

27. Swan HJ, Ganz W, Forrester J, et al. Catheterization of the heart in man with use of a flow-directed balloon-tipped catheter. N Engl J Med 1970;283(9):447–51.

28. Gore JM, Goldberg RJ, Spodick DH, et al. A community-wide assessment of the use of pulmonary artery catheters in patients with acute myocardial infarction. Chest 1987;92(4):721–7.

29. Connors AF, Speroff T, Dawson NV, et al. The effectiveness of right heart catheterization in the initial care of critically ill patients. SUPPORT Investigators. JAMA 1996;276(11):889–97.

30. Sangkum L, Liu GL, Yu L, et al. Minimally invasive or noninvasive cardiac output measurement: an update. J Anesth 2016;30(3):461–80.

31. Pugsley J, Lerner AB. Cardiac output monitoring: is there a gold standard and how do the newer technologies compare? Semin Cardiothorac Vasc Anesth 2010;14(4):274–82.

32. Goedje O, Hoeke K, Lichtwarck-Aschoff M, et al. Continuous cardiac output by femoral arterial thermodilution calibrated pulse contour analysis: comparison with pulmonary arterial thermodilution. Crit Care Med 1999;27(11):2407–12.

33. Tibby SM, Hatherill M, Marsh MJ, et al. Clinical validation of cardiac output measurements using femoral artery thermodilution with direct Fick in ventilated children and infants. Intensive Care Med 1997;23(9):987–91.

34. Buhre W, Weyland A, Kazmaier S, et al. Comparison of cardiac output assessed by pulse-contour analysis and thermodilution in patients undergoing minimally invasive direct coronary artery bypass grafting. J Cardiothorac Vasc Anesth 1999;13(4): 437–40.

35. Linton R, Band D, O'Brien T, et al. Lithium dilution cardiac output measurement: a comparison with thermodilution. Crit Care Med 1997;25(11):1796–800.

36. Reuter DA, Huang C, Edrich T, et al. Cardiac output monitoring using indicator-dilution techniques: basics, limits, and perspectives. Anesth Analg 2010; 110(3):799–811.

37. Ostergaard D, Engbaek J, Viby-Mogensen J. Adverse reactions and interactions of the neuromuscular blocking drugs. Med Toxicol Adverse Drug Exp 1989;4(5):351–68.

38. Pearse RM, Ikram K, Barry J. Equipment review: an appraisal of the LiDCO plus method of measuring cardiac output. Crit Care 2004;8(3):190–5.

39. Costa MG, Della Rocca G, Chiarandini P, et al. Continuous and intermittent cardiac output measurement in hyperdynamic conditions: pulmonary artery catheter vs. lithium dilution technique. Intensive Care Med 2008;34(2):257–63.

40. Hadian M, Kim HK, Severyn DA, et al. Cross-comparison of cardiac output trending accuracy of LiDCO, PiCCO, FloTrac and pulmonary artery catheters. Crit Care 2010;14(6):R212.

41. Mayer J, Boldt J, Poland R, et al. Continuous arterial pressure waveform-based cardiac output using the FloTrac/Vigileo: a review and meta-analysis. J Cardiothorac Vasc Anesth 2009;23(3):401–6.

42. De Backer D, Ospina-Tascon G, Salgado D, et al. Monitoring the microcirculation in the critically ill patient: current methods and future approaches. Intensive Care Med 2010;36(11):1813–25.

43. Desebbe O, Henaine R, Keller G, et al. Ability of the third-generation FloTrac/Vigileo software to track changes in cardiac output in cardiac surgery patients: a polar plot approach. J Cardiothorac Vasc Anesth 2013;27(6):1122–7.

44. Kusaka Y, Yoshitani K, Irie T, et al. Clinical comparison of an echocardiograph-derived versus pulse counter-derived cardiac output measurement in abdominal aortic aneurysm surgery. J Cardiothorac Vasc Anesth 2012;26(2):223–6.

45. Biancofiore G, Critchley LAH, Lee A, et al. Evaluation of an uncalibrated arterial pulse contour cardiac output monitoring system in cirrhotic patients undergoing liver surgery. Br J Anaesth 2009;102(1):47–54.

46. Bogert LWJ, Wesseling KH, Schraa O, et al. Pulse contour cardiac output derived from non-invasive arterial pressure in cardiovascular disease. Anaesthesia 2010;65(11):1119–25.

47. Stover JF, Stocker R, Lenherr R, et al. Noninvasive cardiac output and blood pressure monitoring cannot replace an invasive monitoring system in critically ill patients. BMC Anesthesiol 2009;9:6.

48. Porhomayon J, El-Solh A, Papadakos P, et al. Cardiac output monitoring devices: an analytic review. Intern Emerg Med 2012;7(2):163–71.

49. McLean A, Yastrebov K. Echocardiography training for the intensivist. Crit Care Resusc 2007;9(4): 319–22.

50. Jensen MB, Sloth E, Larsen KM, et al. Transthoracic echocardiography for cardiopulmonary monitoring in intensive care. Eur J Anaesthesiol 2004;21(9): 700–7.

51. Boyd JH, Forbes J, Nakada T, et al. Fluid resuscitation in septic shock: a positive fluid balance and elevated central venous pressure are associated with increased mortality. Crit Care Med 2011;39(2): 259–65.

52. Kanji HD, McCallum J, Sirounis D, et al. Limited echocardiography-guided therapy in subacute shock is associated with change in management and improved outcomes. J Crit Care 2014;29(5): 700–5.

53. Kumar A, Anel R, Bunnell E, et al. Pulmonary artery occlusion pressure and central venous pressure fail to predict ventricular filling volume, cardiac performance, or the response to volume infusion in normal subjects. Crit Care Med 2004;32(3):691–9.

54. Marik PE, Monnet X, Teboul J-L. Hemodynamic parameters to guide fluid therapy. Ann Intensive Care 2011;1(1):1.

55. Bednarczyk JM, Fridfinnson JA, Kumar A, et al. Incorporating dynamic assessment of fluid responsiveness into goal-directed therapy: a systematic review and meta-analysis. Crit Care Med 2017;45(9): 1538–45.

56. Chaves RCF, Corrêa TD, Neto AS, et al. Assessment of fluid responsiveness in spontaneously breathing patients: a systematic review of literature. Ann Intensive Care 2018;8(1):21.

57. Berger MM, Gradwohl-Matis I, Brunauer A, et al. Targets of perioperative fluid therapy and their effects on postoperative outcome: a systematic review and meta-analysis. Minerva Anestesiol 2015;81(7): 794–808.

Advances in Surgical Training Using Simulation

Kamal F. Busaidy, BDS (Lond), FDSRCS (Eng)

KEYWORDS

- Simulation technology • Residency education • Competency assessment
- Oral and maxillofacial surgery

KEY POINTS

- Simulation technology presents key benefits in modern health care education.
- Recent advances in simulation technology have given rise to new applications for simulation-based learning in oral and maxillofacial surgery.
- Modern day learners are receptive to simulation as a tool for learning.
- As mounting research data accumulate to support the validity of simulation in the assessment of competency, stake holders are starting to use simulation for credentialing and licensing pathways.

INTRODUCTION

In the context of health care and health-related education, simulation involves the recreation of real-life situations, processes, or structures for the purpose of improving safety, effectiveness, and efficiency of health care services.[1] In essence, simulation provides a controlled and safe environment for training and assessment. In an age in which regulatory burdens, fiscal challenges, and renewed focus on patient safety increasingly constrain surgical residency programs, innovation in teaching is vital for the future of oral and maxillofacial surgery (OMS) training. Combined with this is the challenge posed by the learning style of the modern trainee. The millennial learner expects to be engaged in the learning process. Information needs to be immediately available and portable. For the modern trainee, doing more is more important than learning more. The Constructivism theory of adult learning, originally espoused by Piaget, holds that students learn best by exploring concepts, generating hypotheses, reflecting on solutions, and experiencing outcomes directly.[2,3] Simulation provides an environment for such exploration, and it facilitates the hands-on experience that modern trainees crave. It is, therefore, an excellent tool through which the modern learner can experience even the rarest event or condition, repeatedly if necessary, to learn more effectively.

Since the dawn of medical education, simulation has had a place in the instruction of trainees in health professions. Cadaver dissection is probably the most vivid example of simulation-based education for the medical and dental student. Dental students have long used a variety of simulation technologies in the course of training, the phantom head being just one example. A variety of modern variations on this theme involve virtual reality (VR) simulators with haptic feedback that enable the operator to prepare teeth in a virtual environment and have that work evaluated, in its digital form, by a faculty member.[4] For the OMS trainee, coming from an educational background where simulation, in its various forms, is so ubiquitous, provides a firm foundation for utilization of simulation technologies in OMS residency training.

Simulation is not a curriculum in and of itself. Rather, it is a tool for teaching a curriculum. A multitude of simulation technologies exist in modern day health care education, many of which have found their way into OMS training. There follows a brief explanation of these technologies, with some examples of their uses in OMS.

Disclosure: The author has nothing to disclose.
Department of Oral and Maxillofacial Surgery, UTHealth-Houston, 7500 Cambridge Street, Suite 6510, Houston, TX 77030, USA
E-mail address: Kamal.Busaidy@uth.tmc.edu

Oral Maxillofacial Surg Clin N Am 31 (2019) 621–626
https://doi.org/10.1016/j.coms.2019.07.006
1042-3699/19/© 2019 Elsevier Inc. All rights reserved.

STANDARDIZED PATIENTS

A standardized patient is one who has been trained to consistently respond in the same way as a real patient with a given medical situation. These live human interactions enable students to practice a broad range of cognitive and noncognitive skills, from history taking and physical examination of a patient, to diagnosis of disease states. Beyond facilitating learning, these encounters are used to facilitate high-stakes assessment of students, such as for licensing examinations, including the US Medical Licensing Examination, part II.[5] However, standardized patients can be expensive because of the amount of training required. This simulation technique has not been previously described in OMS residency training; however, in dental schools, the use of standardized patients has demonstrated benefit in the development of communication skills.[6–8]

VIRTUAL PATIENTS

OMS training frequently involves discussion of cases in a small-group format, with the aim of exploring diagnostic and therapeutic strategies. Virtual patients are cases that are presented in absentia of a real patient. This Socratic approach may use real cases or fabricated cases. Although the format for this presentation can be on paper, these cases have become increasingly elaborate, incorporating digital presentations, and even automated interactivity, such that a facilitator is no longer required for an individual to gain feedback from the exercise.[9] One example of such autonomous learning technology is the use of virtual cases for training and self-assessment in Pediatric Advanced Life Support and Advanced Cardiac Life Support.[10]

TASK TRAINERS

Task trainers are devices designed to facilitate mastery of specific skills. A common example of a task trainer in dental training is the phantom head, which serves as a platform for practicing a variety of different skills before applying them in human patients. In OMS, there are a limited number of task trainers available. Certainly the cheaper modalities are more ubiquitous, but more elaborate varieties can be found on the market. It is not clear how widespread these are being used. Examples of simple task trainers in OMS include suture boards for practicing knot-tying, sawbone skulls for practicing rigid internal fixation, rat models for practicing microvascular anastomosis,[11] and pigs feet for practicing wound closure.

Many OMS programs use task trainers for basic surgical and bedside skills training. At the author's program, first-year residents are required to attend a half-day simulation course practicing tasks such as placement of a Foley catheter, central line placement, intraosseous line placement, nasogastric tube placement, direct laryngoscopy, fiberoptic intubation, and emergency cricothyroidotomy. In addition, they have an opportunity to practice physical diagnosis skills on task trainers specifically designed for those purposes, such as fundoscopy and otoscopy.

More elaborate (and potentially expensive) task trainers for OMS have been developed, but have not yet gained widespread use. Recently published preliminary validation studies for a task trainer designed to simulate the harvesting of an outer table graft from the calvarium, confirmed the realistic experience that can be afforded to the trainees.[12] In another example, a model was developed with 3-dimensional and tactile characteristics similar to human tissues, for the purpose of practicing temporomandibular joint (TMJ) arthroscopy and arthrocentesis. In this example, the developers designed the individual tissues to mimic human tissues in order to closely replicate the sensation of operating through skin, muscle, TMJ capsule, and so forth. Given that each model typically serves to provide one surgical experience before it requires replacement, these task trainers can be expensive. Yet another task trainer was recently developed in Germany for the simulation of radial forearm flap harvesting,[13] and others for teaching early interventions in the management of patients with cleft lip and palate.[14,15]

HIGH-FIDELITY MANIKINS

High-fidelity manikins provide a wide range of options for training OMS residents.[16] This technology incorporates a full-size manikin with lifelike physiologic functions that can be manipulated at a remote computer, by a faculty facilitator, to suit desired training goals (**Fig. 1**). The physiologic functions of the high-fidelity manikin include, for example, heart sounds, blood pressure, palpable pulse, electrocardiogram rhythm, breath sounds, ventilatory chest excursions, and bowel sounds.[17–19] Conditions that can be simulated include numerous cardiac dysrhythmias, diaphoresis, bronchospasm, laryngospasm, trismus, pneumothorax, hypoventilation, hypercarbia, nausea/vomiting, hypertension, hypotension, and anaphylaxis. These capabilities make high-fidelity manikins ideal for training of OMS residents in the management of anesthesia-related emergencies,[16] particularly because uncommon

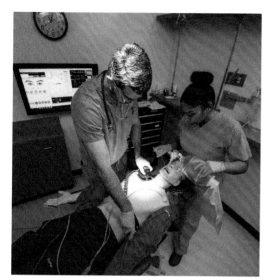

Fig. 1. An OMS resident practices emergency response protocols using a high-fidelity manikin in a simulated scenario.

emergencies can be recreated on demand to facilitate deliberate practice. The myriad of interventions that can be demonstrated on these manikins include peripheral venous catheterization, intraosseous line placement, chest compressions, mask ventilation, endotracheal intubation, fiberoptic intubation, retrograde intubation, cricothyroidotomy, nasogastric tube placement, defibrillation, and cardioversion. Because experiences with a high-fidelity simulator can vary widely, debriefing of participants by a content expert, after each simulation, is critical to facilitate focused reflection and guided learning. Two main drawbacks of this technology include the equipment costs and the training that is required for teaching faculty to learn to control the manikin. These drawbacks can be mitigated to some extent by training midlevel providers for control of the manikin and oversight of the simulation facility, and sharing cost and time in the simulator between departments.[20]

VIRTUAL REALITY

VR uses computer graphics to create a 3-dimensional world in which individuals interact with objects or with each other. The images can be displayed on a computer desktop. However, if the user wears goggles to visualize the virtual world, it is possible to achieve more complete immersion. The realism of the graphical representation of the virtual world is limited by computing power, and it often appears more animated than realistic. Nevertheless, flight simulators that use VR in the aviation industry are an example of VR

that is highly immersive, and have yielded important advances in safety of pilot performance and crisis resource management.[21] VR is often combined with haptic technology to recreate touch sensation by applying forces or vibrations to the user through a joystick or similar handheld device.[22] The addition of touch sensation enables a participant to interact with the virtual environment rather than simply viewing it. VR combined with haptics has been used in dental training to replace phantom heads in the preclinical instruction of dental cavity preparation[4]; however, the sensations generated are not yet fully lifelike and the addition of haptic feedback adds further cost to an already expensive system. Nevertheless, with the explosion in the development of this technology, similar applications are now being used in a variety of medical fields, for training students in spinal needle insertion, ventriculostomy placement, orthopedic fracture reduction, and others.

In OMS, several applications of VR now exist, although many are still in the developmental stages:

- Orthognathic surgery
  Experiences of novice residents were evaluated after using a VR program to view a Le Fort 1 osteotomy, and were compared with 2-dimensional videos and PowerPoint presentations of the same procedure.[23] In the VR program, the residents were able to interact with the skull model to better understand how the mobilized segment related to the skull base. The residents had greater confidence and understanding of the procedure after using the VR program.
- Facial trauma
  Haptic feedback combined with computer-aided simulation has been shown to improve virtual fracture reduction planning and more closely approximate clinical results obtained.[24]
- Dental implants
  A patient-specific haptic drilling simulator based on VR allows trainees to practice implant drilling protocols and even rehearse surgery for a specific patient.[25] This type of "patient-specific simulation" technology is dealt with in the article by Michael F. Huang and colleagues' article, "The Use of Patient-Specific Implants in Oral and Maxillofacial Surgery," elsewhere in this issue.
- Endoscopic removal of submandibular gland
  VR combined with haptic feedback has been developed to teach endoscopic

removal of the submandibular gland. Trainees who underwent training with this system experienced reduced procedure time and a reduced number of errors.[26]

- Local anesthetic delivery
  - VR with haptic feedback has been developed for simulation of inferior alveolar nerve blocks. Student users reported that the experience was very close to reality and improved their confidence in delivery of local anesthetic to patients; however, they also reported that feedback sensation from the haptic device required more refinement.[27]

AUGMENTED REALITY

Augmented reality (AR) uses computer graphics to overlay objects onto what a user sees in the real world. As distinct from VR, in which the user sees a completely fabricated world, in AR the user sees the real environment through a pair of goggles, and the superimposition of images on top of that environment can be used to increase the amount of information available to the user. The superimposed information can be used to inform the user about real structures in view; for example, by superimposing single-photon emission computed tomography images onto the neck of a patient undergoing sentinel lymph node biopsy for treatment of head and neck cancer,[28] or by superimposing patient-specific skeletal images onto a patient's face during orthognathic surgery, to improve orientation of the surgeon.[29] Alternatively, the superimposed information can be used to introduce virtual objects into the real environment; for example, to simulate the presence of an animal in the room in order to safely desensitize a patient with animal phobias.[30] In OMS, AR has been used successfully to provide surgical trainees with the virtual presence of a proctor during surgical management of cleft lip deformities. The system allows experienced surgeons to "virtually" scrub in and teach trainees, introducing their hands and instruments into the trainee's surgical field, even when those trainees were in remote locations.[31]

SERIOUS GAMES

Most teenagers are familiar with the concept of playing games for entertainment; however, recent developments in "serious games" have led to the application of play as a tool for engaging learners to improve knowledge acquisition, advance decision-making skills and coordination, and increase levels of motivation. This approach has been applied to education and training in fields such as the military, engineering, computing, and health care,[32,33] although there has not been any description of serious games applied to OMS as yet.

SIMULATION-BASED PERFORMANCE ASSESSMENT

Simulation, in its many various forms described previously, has been used for assessment of students and practitioners for decades. As a tool for formative assessment, there is little argument that it provides many advantages (**Box 1**). However, as a tool for high-stakes assessment in licensing or maintenance of certification, the use of simulation requires that validated rubrics and standard setting be established before considering the logistics of administering assessments on a broad basis.

Several medical specialty boards have opted to use simulation-based assessment as part of their initial licensing or maintenance of certification standards:

- The American Board of Surgery requires graduating residents to have passed a simulation-based Fundamentals of Laparoscopic Surgery test (FLS). FLS is a comprehensive Web-based education module that includes a hands-on skills training component and assessment tool designed to teach the physiology, fundamental knowledge, and technical skills required in basic laparoscopic surgery.[34]

Box 1
Advantages of simulation-based learning in health care

- Customized learning experiences: The content and complexity of the curriculum can be tailored to the specific learner. Episodes of learning can be scheduled so as to avoid conflicts in patient care and other responsibilities.

- Deliberate practice: The learner can repeat simulations with intentional focus on correcting areas of weakness until mastery has been achieved.

- Safe environment: Patients are not put at risk when trainees practice in a simulated environment. Learners have the freedom to make mistakes and learn from them.

- Building self-confidence: Students are more confident in managing patients when they first practice procedures in a simulated environment.

- The American Board of Family Medicine requires physicians to undergo computer-based Knowledge Self-Assessment and Clinical Simulation Assessment modules as part of initial certification and maintenance of certification.[35]
- The American Board of Anesthesiology recently introduced a requirement for new licensees to pass an Objective Structured Clinical Examination, focusing on communication, professionalism, critical thinking, ethics, interpretation of monitors, and technical skills.[36] High-fidelity simulation remains an option for satisfying the Quality Improvement component of the Maintenance of Certification in Anesthesia.

The American Association of Oral and Maxillofacial Surgery recently funded the development of a series of simulation-based programs related to emergencies during outpatient anesthesia. The series involves Basic Emergency Airway Management, Office-Based Crisis Management, and Intravenous Sedation. Following a rigorous period of data collection and validation of the assessment rubrics and performance standards expected within the program, the first of these modules was offered to attendees at the 2018 annual American Association of Oral and Maxillofacial Surgeons meeting. Although the course is not currently mandatory, the intention is that these programs will form the basis for the introduction of objective simulation-based performance assessments, perhaps as part of the Office Anesthesia Evaluation, in the future.[37]

SUMMARY

Simulation-based training in health care education is not new, although recent advances in high-fidelity approaches to simulation have ignited a surge in applications for health care training. As simulation technology advances, applications specific to OMS also are expanding. Simulation-based assessment for measurement of competency is the latest focus of agencies and professional associations. As validation data for these assessment modalities improve, increasing attention from stake holders will inevitably bring mandates for incorporation of simulation-based assessment into licensing and credentialing pathways in the future.[38]

REFERENCES

1. SSH. About Simulation. 2019. Available at: https://www.ssih.org/About-SSH/About-Simulation. Accessed May 6, 2019.
2. Newcombe NS. Cognitive development: changing views of cognitive change. Wiley Interdiscip Rev Cogn Sci 2013;4(5):479–91.
3. Fosnot CT, editor. Constructivism: theory, perspectives and practice. 2nd edition. New York: Teachers College, Columbia University; 2005.
4. Roy E, Bakr MM, George R. The need for virtual reality simulators in dental education: A review. Saudi Dent J 2017;29(2):41–7.
5. Boulet JR, Smee SM, Dillon GF, et al. The use of standardized patient assessments for certification and licensure decisions. Simul Healthc 2009;4(1):35–42.
6. McKenzie CT, Tilashalski KR, Peterson DT, et al. Effectiveness of standardized patient simulations in teaching clinical communication skills to dental students. J Dent Educ 2017;81(10):1179–86.
7. Johnson JA, Kopp KC, Williams RG. Standardized patients for the assessment of dental students' clinical skills. J Dent Educ 1990;54(6):331–3.
8. Broder HL, Janal M. Promoting interpersonal skills and cultural sensitivity among dental students. J Dent Educ 2006;70(4):409–16.
9. Kishimoto N, Mukai N, Honda Y, et al. Simulation training for medical emergencies in the dental setting using an inexpensive software application. Eur J Dent Educ 2018;22(3):e350–7.
10. AHA. Pediatric advanced life support elearning course. 2019. Availabe at: https://elearning.heart.org/course/22. Accessed January 12, 2019.
11. Shurey S, Akelina Y, Legagneux J, et al. The rat model in microsurgery education: classical exercises and new horizons. Arch Plast Surg 2014;41(3):201–8.
12. Hollensteiner M, Malek M, Augat P, et al. Validation of a simulator for cranial graft lift training: face, content, and construct validity. J Craniomaxillofac Surg 2018;46(8):1390–4.
13. Nobis CP, Bauer F, Rohleder NH, et al. Development of a haptic model for teaching in reconstructive surgery—the radial forearm flap. Simul Healthc 2014;9(3):203–8.
14. Rau A, Nobis CP, Behr AV, et al. Design of a haptic model for the training of cleft treatment procedures. Simul Healthc 2015;10(2):128–32.
15. Cote V, Schwartz M, Arbouin Vargas JF, et al. 3-Dimensional printed haptic simulation model to teach incomplete cleft palate surgery in an international setting. Int J Pediatr Otorhinolaryngol 2018;113:292–7.
16. Hassan ZU, D'Addario M, Sloan PA. Human patient simulator for training oral and maxillofacial surgery residents in general anesthesia and airway management. J Oral Maxillofac Surg 2007;65(9):1892–7.
17. Gaumard. Available at: https://www.gaumard.com/products/tetherless/hal. Accessed January 21, 2019.
18. Laerdal. Available at: https://www.laerdal.com/us/doc/85/SimMan-3G. Accessed January 21, 2019.

19. CAE. Available at: https://caehealthcare.com/patient-simulation/apollo/. Accessed January 21, 2019.

20. Edler AA, Chen M, Honkanen A, et al. Affordable simulation for small-scale training and assessment. Simul Healthc 2010;5(2):112–5.

21. Kanki BG, Anca J, Chidester T. Crew resource management. 3rd edition. San Diego (CA): Academic Press; 2019.

22. 3D-Systems. Available at: https://www.3dsystems.com/scanners-haptics - haptics-devices?utm_source=geomagic.com&utm_medium=301. Accessed January 22, 2019.

23. Pulijala Y, Ma M, Pears M, et al. Effectiveness of immersive virtual reality in surgical training—a randomized control trial. J Oral Maxillofac Surg 2018;76(5):1065–72.

24. Girod S, Schvartzman SC, Gaudilliere D, et al. Haptic feedback improves surgeons' user experience and fracture reduction in facial trauma simulation. J Rehabil Res Dev 2016;53(5):561–70.

25. Chen X, Sun P, Liao D. A patient-specific haptic drilling simulator based on virtual reality for dental implant surgery. Int J Comput Assist Radiol Surg 2018;13(11):1861–70.

26. Miki T, Iwai T, Kotani K, et al. Development of a virtual reality training system for endoscope-assisted submandibular gland removal. J Craniomaxillofac Surg 2016;44(11):1800–5.

27. Correa CG, Machado M, Ranzini E, et al. Virtual reality simulator for dental anesthesia training in the inferior alveolar nerve block. J Appl Oral Sci 2017;25(4):357–66.

28. Profeta AC, Schilling C, McGurk M. Augmented reality visualization in head and neck surgery: an overview of recent findings in sentinel node biopsy and future perspectives. Br J Oral Maxillofac Surg 2016;54(6):694–6.

29. Badiali G, Ferrari V, Cutolo F, et al. Augmented reality as an aid in maxillofacial surgery: validation of a wearable system allowing maxillary repositioning. J Craniomaxillofac Surg 2014;42(8):1970–6.

30. Botella C, Perez-Ara MA, Breton-Lopez J, et al. In vivo versus augmented reality exposure in the treatment of small animal phobia: a randomized controlled trial. PLoS One 2016;11(2):e0148237.

31. Vyas R, Bendit D, Hamdan U. Using virtual augmented reality to remotely proctor international cleft surgery: building long-term capacity and sustainability. Cleft Palate Craniofac J 2016;53(4):E102.

32. Sipiyaruk K, Gallagher JE, Hatzipanagos S, et al. A rapid review of serious games: from healthcare education to dental education. Eur J Dent Educ 2018;22(4):243–57.

33. Graafland M, Vollebergh MF, Lagarde SM, et al. A serious game can be a valid method to train clinical decision-making in surgery. World J Surg 2014;38(12):3056–62.

34. FLS. Fundamentals of laparoscopic surgery. Available at: https://www.flsprogram.org/. Accessed January 30, 2019.

35. ABFM. Available at: https://www.theabfm.org/cert/index.aspx. Accessed January 30, 2019.

36. ABA. The American Board of Anesthesiology APPLIED (staged) examination. Available at: http://www.theaba.org/Exams/APPLIED-(Staged-Exam)/About-APPLIED-(Staged-Exam). Accessed January 30, 2019.

37. Todd DW, Schaefer JJ 3rd. The American Association of oral and maxillofacial surgeons simulation program. Oral Maxillofac Surg Clin North Am 2018;30(2):195–206.

38. Boulet JR. Summative assessment in medicine: the promise of simulation for high-stakes evaluation. Acad Emerg Med 2008;15(11):1017–24.

Advances in Functional Imaging in the Assessment of Head and Neck Cancer

David Q. Wan, MD

KEYWORDS

- FDG PET/CT • Head and neck cancer • Ga-68 DOTATATE PET/CT • Neuroendocrine tumor
- Paraganglioma

KEY POINTS

- PET/CT with fludeoxyglucose (FDG PET/CT) imaging interpretation to differentiate head and neck cancer recurrence from posttreatment changes.
- FDG PET/CT imaging allows for the localization of nearly half of unknown primary tumor sites not detectable by traditional imaging.
- A negative posttreatment FDG PET/CT scan is a reliable sign of good prognosis.
- Patients with head and neck cancer need to follow specific preparation and imaging protocols.
- Gallium-68 DOTATATE PET/CT is a new test for neuroendocrine tumor.

INTRODUCTION

The trend of functional molecular imaging has largely shifted to Positron Emission Tomography (PET). PET imaging is superior to traditional nuclear medicine scans, such as single-photon emission tomography (SPECT). Over the past 2 decades, newer and more advanced positron emitters have been developed and even more molecules have been linked to those positron radiotracers for various purposes. To this date, the Food and Drug Administration (FDA) has approved at least 6 different types of PET scans for clinical use, including Fluorine 18 FDG and, more recently, Gallium-68 (Ga-68) DOTATATE for neuroendocrine tumors. FDG PET/computed tomography (CT) is by far the most useful scan in both oncology and neurology. This article reviews FDG PET/CT scan applications for head and neck cancer and provides a brief introduction to the Ga-68 DOTATATE PET/CT scan for neuroendocrine tumors.

FDG PET/CT FOR HEAD AND NECK CANCER, INITIAL DIAGNOSIS AND STAGING

Currently, CT and MRI scans remain as the first-line diagnostic tools for head and neck cancer diagnosis and initial staging given their high resolution and detailed anatomy, which are critical for surgical planning. The FDG PET/CT scan is complementary to contrast CT and MRI scans during initial diagnosis and staging.[1] FDG PET/CT is especially useful for the localization of an unknown primary tumor site in a patient with a positive cervical lymph node metastasis by biopsy but with an undetectable primary tumor by conventional CT or MRI. Nearly half (26%–56%) of head and neck squamous carcinomas that initially present as an unknown primary by conventional examination of CT/MRI, can be detected by FDG PET/CT scan[2,3] (**Fig. 1**).

Disclosure Statement: The author has nothing to disclose.
Department of Diagnostic and Interventional Imaging, McGovern Medical School, Health Science Center in Houston, University of Texas, MSB 2.130B, 6431 Fannin Street, Houston, TX 77030, USA
E-mail address: david.q.wan@uth.tmc.edu

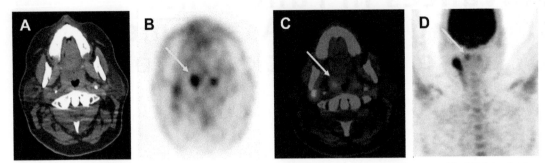

Fig. 1. Contrast CT image of a 42-year-old woman with squamous cell carcinoma discovered by biopsy of a 2-cm right cervical lymph node, but with no clear primary tumor lesion identified by CT (*A*). FDG PET axial projection (*B*), PET and CT fused image (*C*) and coronal maximum intensity projection (MIP) image (*D*) showed asymmetric focal FDG uptake (*yellow arrow*) in the right tonsil. Subsequent surgical pathology proved this to be the primary tumor site. Please note that the PET-only image (*B*) showed a clearer asymmetric uptake in right tonsil compared with the PET and CT fused image (*C*).

FDG PET/CT COMPARED WITH CONTRAST CT AND MRI

CT and MRI imaging rely on a pattern of contrast enhancement and sizing criteria to differentiate tumor involvement from normal tissue, which are both nonspecific. In the head and neck region, contrast enhancement is especially unreliable because of normal tissue enhancement of the tongue, tonsils, mucosa, thyroid, and reactive lymph nodes. Early lymph node metastases may be smaller than 1 cm in diameter, which would be interpreted as benign using CT or MRI standards. FDG PET/CT is superior to contrast-enhanced CT scan for the staging of regional metastatic disease with higher sensitivity (87% vs 62%) and specificity (89% vs 73%).[4] In the oral cavity, FDG PET/CT is also superior to CT or MRI for primary tumor detection with a sensitivity of 96.3% compared with 77.8% for CT and 85.2% for MRI.[5] This is largely due to the high frequency of patients with dental hardware producing more artifact on CT and MRI images than on PET images (**Fig. 2**). FDG PET/CT has another advantage over CT or MRI in the detection of distant metastasis (**Fig. 3**) or in

patients who have a second primary tumor (**Fig. 4**). The finding of a concurrent second primary cancer, mostly in the lungs, is not uncommon in head and neck cancer patients, especially for those who smoke. In up to 15% of patients with squamous cell carcinoma of the head and neck, FDG PET/CT may identify a second primary tumor with high accuracy of 82%.[6]

POSTTREATMENT ASSESSMENT AND PATIENT FOLLOW-UP

FDG PET relies on glucose metabolic activity to assess cellular function, and this can be used to detect treatment response at an earlier time point compared with anatomic imaging. Tumor cell injury as a result of therapy will be detected through its altered intracellular glucose mechanism by FDG PET scan before structural changes, such as decreased tumor size, which are detected by anatomic imaging of CT or MRI. Normally, the FDG PET scan is able to detect a tumor response to therapy within weeks, compared with anatomic imaging techniques, which can take months. FDG PET/CT has also proven to have a significant

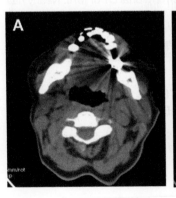
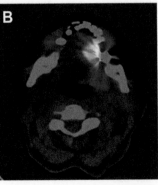

Fig. 2. Axial CT (*A*) and PET CT fused images (*B*) for staging of a 71-year-old man with left gingival cancer. Dental hardware prevents detailed examination on CT. PET images show a clear focal area of tracer uptake to suggest tumor involvement.

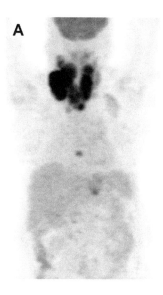

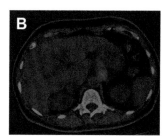

Fig. 3. Coronal PET (*A*) and axial PET CT fused (*B*) images of a 72-year-old man with laryngeal cancer and distant nodal mediastinal metastasis and left adrenal metastasis.

advantage over traditional imaging techniques with respect to the restaging of patients after chemotherapy or radiotherapy. Prognosis is excellent for patients who have had a complete response to therapy as shown on FDG PET/CT scans.[7] The negative predictive value (97%) of FDG PET/CT following treatment is extremely accurate.[8,9]

POTENTIAL FALSE-POSITIVE FDG PET/CT SCAN IN RESTAGING PATIENTS WITH HEAD AND NECK CANCER

Despite the utility and advantages of FDG PET scanning, interpretation of a positive posttreatment scan may present some challenges. An FDG PET/CT scan is not a tumor-specific scan. It detects cellular glucose uptake activity during normal and other pathologic states, such as uptake by contracting muscle cells, by lymphocytes during inflammation, or by leukocytes during infection.

FDG uptake can occur in postsurgical wound inflammation (lasting for at least 1 month for oral or nasopharyngeal surgery) or in an infected surgical wound in which the activity duration would be longer. It also can occur in postradiation inflammation (lasting at least 2 months), as physiologic uptake in muscles (most often the masseter or pterygoid muscles during mastication, the longus capitis when turning the neck, and the tongue/vocal cords when speaking), in the tonsils after an upper-respiratory infection, and physiologic uptake in the salivary glands.

A FEW POINTS TO CONSIDER WHEN READING A HEAD AND NECK FDG PET/CT IMAGE

Because of the common occurrence of nonspecific FDG uptake in the oral and nasopharyngeal regions, FDG PET/CT image interpretation can be complicated. When considering a true tumor recurrence, the following must be considered:

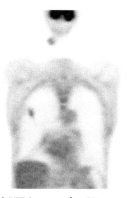

Fig. 4. Coronal PET image of a 65-year-old man with right laryngeal cancer for initial staging showed a solitary FDG avid right lung nodule. The radiology report stated a possible second primary lung cancer, because of the single dominant lesion in the lung and smoking history. Metastasis from laryngeal cancer is less likely but not excluded. Biopsy of the lung nodule proved to be primary lung cancer. The staging for both cancers was changed and the treatment plan was altered accordingly.

a. *Focal in appearance* (**Fig. 5**). Generally, cancer appears as focal uptake that is best illustrated on PET-only images, rather than PET and CT fused images that interfere with each other's image quality (see **Figs. 1**B, C and **5**D, E). FDG uptake at postradiation inflammatory sites usually appears hazy, blurred, and nonfocal (**Fig. 6**).

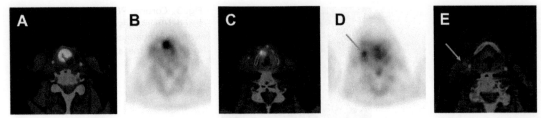

Fig. 5. Axial PET CT fused initial staging image (*A*) of a 62-year-old woman with right laryngeal cancer. The PET axial image (*B*) and PET CT fused image (*C*) of a post radiation therapy restaging scan demonstrates a small focal uptake in the right vocal cord at the exact site of primary lesion (*A*), consistent with residual disease. There is another small focal uptake nearby on the same side of the primary lesion which was proven to be a 6-mm nodal metastasis (*blue arrows*). This positive node was initially identified on the PET-only image (*D*) with better contrast over background compared with the PET CT fused image (*E*).

b. *The geographic location of the lesion.* In general, if a suspicious area of FDG activity is distant from the primary tumor site and not in an area of lymph nodes, the likelihood of tumor being recurrence is small. If the primary lesion crosses the midline, a suspicion for a contralateral tumor metastasis would be high (**Fig. 7**). The presence or absence of contralateral disease affects presurgical planning and should be evaluated in every head and neck PET/CT examination.

c. *Time since most recent chemotherapy or radiation therapy.* From the author's experience, head and neck squamous cell carcinomas that show a complete response to treatment by FDG PET/CT rarely reoccur within 1 year. Postradiation inflammation can last from months to years. Generally, increased uptake will occur within 2 months, whereas decreased uptake is seen after 6 months, given no secondary infection occurs. Asymmetric activity in paired bilateral organs (tonsils, salivary glands, thyroid, and muscles) after radiation can be confusing because the contralateral nonradiated healthy side will show relatively increased uptake and may

be incorrectly diagnosed as recurrence (**Figs. 8** and **9**).

d. *Comparison with a previous scan.* Cancers grow in size over time. A lesion that shows high FDG uptake (high glucose requirement) but stabilizes in size over time, is likely benign provided that no recent antitumor therapy was given. Cellular glucose consumption in such benign lesions is for functional activity rather than cellular growth. In contrast, a lesion that demonstrates interval increased, stable, or even decreased but persistent FDG uptake and growth in size could be cancer.

e. *Follow-up scan.* When a suspected lesion is encountered for the first time and is difficult to characterize, a follow-up FDG PET/CT scan is recommended to monitor both the metabolic activity and size of the lesion. Generally speaking, the higher the FDG uptake, the less time is needed to verify the nature of the lesion. In the author's experience, when the measured lesion Ideal Body Weight corrected Standard Uptake Value (SUV) is higher than 5, a 3-month to 6-month follow-up is sufficient. If the SUV is less than 3, the follow-up time would be extended to 6 to

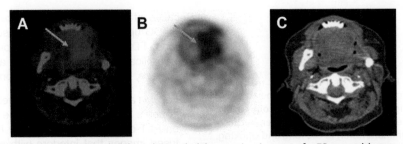

Fig. 6. Axial PET CT fused (*A*), PET-only (*B*), and CT-only (*C*) restaging images of a 58-year-old man with right-sided cancer at the base of the tongue 3 months after radiation therapy. There is resolved FDG uptake in the primary lesion on the right side of the tongue, suggesting good response to therapy. However, there is new mild hazy FDG uptake on the left side of the tongue (*arrows*) without corresponding soft tissue swelling on CT image. The activity resolved on a follow-up scan taken 1 year later and was consistent with post radiation inflammation.

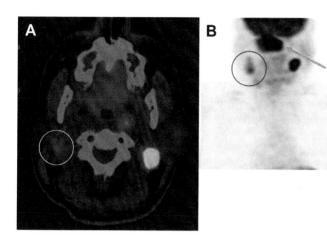

Fig. 7. Axial PET CT fused (A) and coronal (B) initial staging images of a 52-year-old man with superior pharyngeal cancer. The primary lesion is located mostly on the left but crosses the mid line (*arrow*). There is intense FDG uptake in an enlarged left cervical node and is consistent with local metastasis. There are mild FDG avid smaller right cervical nodes (*circle*). Considering the location of the primary lesion, the right cervical nodes were considered metastases and biopsy was recommended. The surgical plan was altered accordingly.

12 months. A malignant lesion should be "double positive" over time, because of glucose intake (PET positive) and growth in size (CT positive). An FDG PET positive and CT negative (no growth over time) lesion is considered benign. An FDG PET negative (no glucose uptake) lesion is benign, regardless of the CT findings.

PATIENT INSTRUCTION AND IMAGING PROTOCOL

a. *Insulin effect*: FDG PET scan is significantly influenced by glucose metabolism. High levels of blood glucose can compete with the radiotracer-labeled glucose and reduce the image sensitivity. However, the key factor affecting the FDG PET scan is the insulin, not the levels of blood glucose. When patients receive an insulin injection or are postprandial with native insulin release, most of the injected radiotracer-labeled glucose will be directed into muscle cells and the liver, resulting in significantly reduced scan sensitivity. With low

sensitivity and a high image background due to peripheral muscular FDG uptake, contrast between the actual lesion and the background is reduced. Most of these scans are marked as nondiagnostic and commonly referred to as a "muscle scan" (**Fig. 10**). In certain circumstances, diabetic patients with very high blood glucose levels can be allowed to proceed for an FDG PET scan because a low-sensitive FDG PET scan would still be informative compared with a nondiagnostic post-insulin release "muscle scan." Rescheduling these types of patients in hopes of a lower glucose level is futile in most cases. Diabetic patients are routinely scheduled as early patients in the morning. These patients are instructed to take insulin during their last supper and to skip any breakfast in the morning.

b. *Radiotracer injection and subsequent incubation time*: Coming to my clinic one day, I witnessed a scene that I will never forget. A patient with head and neck cancer was talking loudly on the cellphone while the technologist attempted to inject the FDG tracer. The action

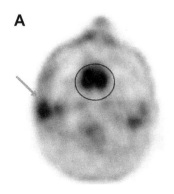
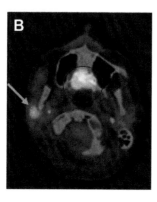

Fig. 8. Axial PET-only (A) and PET CT fused (B) images of a 54-year-old man with right pharyngeal cancer 2 months after radiation. The primary cancer is now essentially undetectable. However, there is new focally asymmetrically increased FDG uptake in the right parotid gland (*arrows*) that resolved on a 1-year follow-up scan, consistent with post radiation inflammation. Symmetric uptake in the soft palate is physiologic in nature (*circles*).

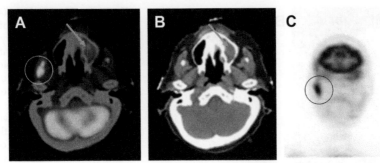

Fig. 9. Axial PET CT fused (*A*), CT-only (*B*), and coronal PET-only (*C*) restaging images of a 63-year-old woman with left nasopharyngeal cancer 2 years post radiation therapy. There is focal cancer recurrence in the left maxillary sinus (*arrows*). There is asymmetric focal physiologic uptake in the right masseter muscle (*circles*) without a corresponding morphologic change on CT. The left masseter muscle does not show uptake secondary to previous radiation damage.

of talking would increase uptake in the tongue and vocal cords, while head movements may cause asymmetric uptake in the longus capitis muscles, all of which can make false-positive findings. Immediately after the tracer injection, patients should be placed in a quiet and dark private room to rest without any interactions from the surroundings.

c. *Special protocols for patients with head and neck cancer*: Although most patients with cancer receive single PET/CT scan imaging protocols, patients with head and neck cancer should receive 2 sets of PET/CT scans. The first is to scan the head and neck areas with the arms down to reduce the attenuation artifact from the arms and to better illustrate the primary lesion and areas of local nodal metastasis

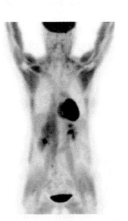

Fig. 10. MIP image of FDG PET scan of a diabetic patient after insulin injection. Small tumors or tumors with low levels of FDG uptake detected by a normal FDG PET scan could be easily missed by this "muscle scan" due to increased background and tracer shifting into muscle. Postprandial (triggering of native insulin release) FDG injection of a nondiabetic patient can cause similar results.

(**Fig. 11**A). The second set of images is a lower body scan with the arms raised to reduce the attenuation artifact from the arms on the lower body and to better survey possible distant metastases below the neck (**Fig. 11**B).

d. *Radiation planning*: FDG PET/CT scans can be performed on an identical table, flat or curved, to ensure accurate imaging for correlation between the PET and CT/MRI data. The patient's position during PET/CT imaging also may be positioned on the radiation treatment table to ensure the exact location of the lesion between the PET scan and the radiation (**Fig. 12**). Another advantage of this technique is to eliminate patient motion artifact by using the radiation fixation mesh. The mesh is necessary for precise positioning during simulation and actual radiation and serves the same purpose during PET/CT scanning.

SUMMARY OF FDG PET/CT ROLES IN HEAD AND NECK CANCER

1. FDG PET/CT technology is outstanding for oral cavity lesions in patients with significant dental artifact shown on CT and MRI scans.[5]
2. FDG PET/CT technology has become essential for the staging and restaging of patients with head and neck cancer and for the evaluation for distant metastasis.[1]
3. Nearly half of the unknown primary head and neck tumors that are undetectable by conventional CT or MRI can be located by FDG PET/CT scans.[2,3]
4. A negative FDG PET/CT scan post treatment is a reliable indicator of a complete response to therapy and excellent prognosis.[7]
5. An FDG PET scan is not a tumor-specific scan, but rather a glucose uptake scan. Not all hot spots are cancers. Noncancerous FDG activity

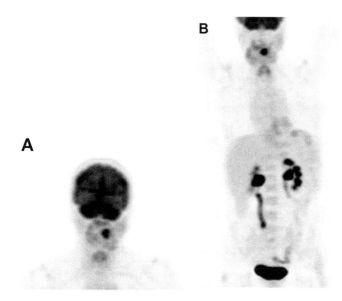

Fig. 11. FDG PET/CT specific protocol for patient with head and neck cancer with 2 sets of images. The first set image of the upper body with arms down (*A*) improves the image quality of head and neck areas with less attenuation artifact from the arms. The second set image of the lower body with the arms up increases the image quality of the lower body for distant metastasis surveying (*B*). The first set image of the upper body and head and neck areas has more clinical value and should be acquired first when patient is less fatigued and able to lie still.

in a post-therapy scan may be confused as residual tumor/recurrence.

6. Preimaging patient instructions and imaging protocol are critical for a successful FDG PET/CT scan.

SOMATOSTATIN RECEPTOR IMAGING WITH GALLIUM-68 DOTATATE PET/CT FOR NEUROENDOCRINE TUMORS, SUCH AS PARAGANGLIOMA
Neuroendocrine Tumors

Paragangliomas originate from embryonic neural crest paraganglia cells of the neuroendocrine system, and function as part of the sympathetic nervous system. These cells generally serve as signal receptors along arteries, commonly in the carotid body and the aortic body. Paragangliomas and pheochromocytomas are closely related neuroendocrine tumors.

Why the New Scan for Neuroendocrine Tumors

Somatostatin is a peptide hormone that regulates hormone secretion and cell proliferation, generally with an inhibitory effect on cell activity. The somatostatin receptor (SSTR) located on neuroendocrine cells bind to somatostatin and this has long been the target for neuroendocrine tumor labeling, traditionally as the indium-111 Octreotide SPECT scan.[10] In 2017, the FDA approved a new PET/CT scan to identify SSTR for neuroendocrine tumors, the ^{68}Ga DOTATATE.

[68]Ga DOTATATE characteristics:

1. [68]Ga is a positron emitter as in a PET scan, which is superior in image quality compared with SPECT scan.
2. [68]Ga has a short half-life of 68 minutes compared with that of Indium 111, which is 2.8 days, resulting in a significant reduction of radiation exposure to patients.
3. [68]Ga DOTATATE scanning requires approximately 1.5 hours to complete compared with 48 to 72 hours for Indium Octreotide SPECT.
4. The new chelating agent (DOTA) and the new somatostatin analogue peptide (TATE) have higher binding affinity to SSTR, especially

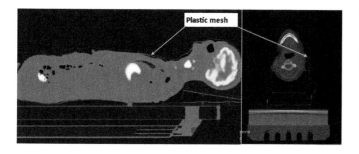

Fig. 12. PET/CT performed on the exact flat radiation table mimicking the fixed position for radiation. The plastic mesh and flat radiation table are necessary for precise positioning during radiation and during PET/CT scanning.

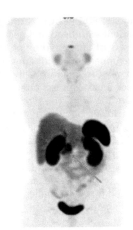

Fig. 13. Normal tracer distribution of the ^{68}Ga DOTATATE scan in pituitary gland, salivary glands, thyroid, liver, spleen, kidneys, bladder and bowel. Physiologic uptake in the pancreatic uncinate process (*arrow*) could be misinterpreted as pathologic as this finding was rarely seen on Octreotide scan.

receptor subtype 2, which is expressed in most neuroendocrine tumors.[11]

The Application of Gallium-68 DOTATATE PET/CT

This scan is superior to conventional imaging modalities for neuroendocrine tumor staging and the localization of unknown primary tumors with a sensitivity of 93% and a specificity of 95%.[12,13] Given the higher affinity of the TATE peptide, the superior image quality of PET, and lower background activity in soft tissue and muscle, ^{68}Ga DOTATATE is now considered as the first-line imaging modality for SSTR-positive tumors.

There is physiologic radiotracer distribution to the pituitary gland, salivary glands, thyroid, liver, spleen, stomach, adrenal medullas, kidneys, bladder, and bowel (**Fig. 13**). Occasionally, there is physiologic uptake in the pancreatic uncinate process, which is usually nonfocal and curvilinear in appearance. The physiologic uptake present in the liver may confound findings; in turn, if a lesion is suspected in the liver, one could suggest an MRI, as it may be more sensitive in detecting liver metastases of neuroendocrine tumors with weak SSTR expression. [68]Ga DOTATATE is highly recommended for paraganglioma because of the high tumor/background contrast in the head and neck region (**Fig. 14**). This scan can identify all neuroendocrine lesions, including medullary thyroid cancer or a parathyroid lesion in the head and neck.

The Complementary Nature of Gallium-68 DOTATATE PET/CT and FDG PET/CT

The better-differentiated neuroendocrine tumors closely resemble their original cells and express higher SSTR, resulting in more sensitive testing with ^{68}Ga DOTATATE, as opposed to poorly differentiated neuroendocrine tumors, which differ from their normal tissue and express less SSTR, resulting in less sensitive ^{68}Ga DOTATATE tests. However, the poorly differentiated tumors proliferate more aggressively, rendering the FDG PET/CT more sensitive for these kinds of tumors. [68]Ga DOTATATE PET/CT and FDG PET/CT are complementary in detecting neuroendocrine tumors with high or low SSTR expression.[14]

Direction for Therapy

Detecting SSTR expression in neuroendocrine tumors is not only important for diagnosis, it is also crucial for directing patient management. SSTR-positive patients with high ^{68}Ga DOTATATE uptake will benefit from somatostatin analogue therapy for symptom control and for its

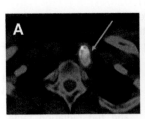
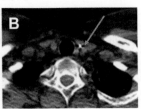
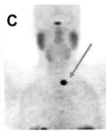

Fig. 14. A 46-year-old woman with headache, intermittent hypertension, and clinical suspicion of pheochromocytoma/paraganglioma. Traditional imaging workup including contrast CT of the chest, abdomen, and pelvis; MRI of brain; and Iodine-123 Metaiodobenzylguanidine (MIBG) scan were all reported as normal. [68]Ga DOTATATE axial images of PET CT fused (*A*), CT-only (*B*) and coronal PET-only (*C*) images clearly identified an intense focus of tracer uptake near the left thoracic inlet, corresponding to a 6-mm soft tissue lesion on CT images (*arrows*). Please note that because of the strong tracer uptake in the lesion and a relatively clear background, the lesion on the PET image appears much larger than it really is because of tracer scattering.

antiproliferative effects. In 2018, the FDA approved a new targeted radionuclide therapy for SSTR-positive tumors by linking the β-emitter Lutetium 177 with Octreotide.[10]

REFERENCES

1. Subramaniam RM, Truong M, Peller P, et al. Fluoro-deoxyglucose-positron-emission tomography imaging of head and neck squamous cell cancer. AJNR Am J Neuroradiol 2010;31:598–604.

2. Rudmik L, Lau HY, Matthews TW, et al. Clinical utility of PET/CT in the evaluation of head and neck squamous cell carcinoma with an unknown primary: a prospective clinical trial. Head Neck 2011;33: 935–40.

3. Miller FR, Hussey D, Beeram M, et al. Positron emission tomography in the management of unknown primary head and neck carcinoma. Arch Otolaryngol Head Neck Surg 2005;131:626–9.

4. Scarfone C, Lavely WC, Cmelak AJ, et al. Prospective feasibility trial of radiotherapy target definition for head and neck cancer using 3-dimensional PET and CT imaging. J Nucl Med 2004;45(4): 543–52.

5. Baek C-H, Chung MK, Son Y-I, et al. Tumor volume assessment by 18F-FDG PET/CT in patients with oral cavity cancer with dental artifacts on CT or MR images. J Nucl Med 2008;49(9): 1422–8.

6. Al-Ibraheem A, Buck A, Krause BJ, et al. Clinical applications of FDG PET and PET/CT in head and neck cancer. J Oncol 2009;2009:208725.

7. Martin RC, Fulham M, Shannon KF, et al. Accuracy of positron emission tomography in the evaluation of patients treated with chemoradiotherapy for mucosal head and neck cancer. Head and Neck 2009;31(2):244–50.

8. Schöder H, Fury M, Lee N, et al. PET monitoring of therapy response in head and neck squamous cell carcinoma. J Nucl Med 2009;50(suppl 1): 74S–88S.

9. Kitagawa Y, Nishizawa S, Sano K. Prospective comparison of 18F-FDG PET with conventional imaging modalities (MRI, CT, and 67Ga scintig-raphy) in assessment of combined intraarterial chemotherapy and radiotherapy for head and neck carcinoma. J Nucl Med 2003;44(2): 198–206.

10. Hicks RJ. Use of molecular targeted agents for the diagnosis, staging and therapy of neuroendocrine malignancy. Cancer Imaging 2010;10(Spec No A): S83–91.

11. Jaïs P, Terris B, Ruszniewski P, et al. Somatostatin receptor subtype gene expression in human endocrine gastroentero-pancreatic tumours. Eur J Clin Invest 1997;27(8):639–44.

12. Geijer H, Breimer LH. Somatostatin receptor PET/CT in neuroendocrine tumours: update on systematic review and meta-analysis. Eur J Nucl Med Mol Imaging 2013;40(11):1770–80.

13. Taïeb D, Timmers HJ, Hindié E, et al. EANM 2012 guidelines for radionuclide imaging of phaeochromocytoma and paraganglioma. Eur J Nucl Med Mol Imaging 2012;39(12): 1977–95.

14. Hofman MS, Hicks RJ. Changing paradigms with molecular imaging of neuroendocrine tumors. Discov Med 2012;14(74):71–81.

Preparation of the Neck for Advanced Flap Reconstruction

Jonathan W. Shum, DDS, MD[a,*], James C. Melville, DDS[a],
Marcus Couey, DDS, MD[b]

KEYWORDS

- Microvascular reconstruction • Neck dissection • Vessel exploration • Microvascular surgery
- Surgical technique

KEY POINTS

- The incorporation of microvascular reconstructions has increased among oral and maxillofacial surgeons.
- Due to the increasing prevalence of advanced flap reconstructions, it is necessary for oral surgeons to be proficient in vascular access and neck vessel preparation to facilitate reconstructions as a 2-teamed approach.
- Vessel preparation is technique sensitive.

INTRODUCTION

The introduction of microvascular reconstruction was among the most significant advances in head and neck surgery in the twentieth century, and continued refinement in these techniques has allowed for reliable reconstruction of virtually any surgical defect of the head and neck.[1] Although many options are available for reconstruction in the maxillofacial region, free tissue transfer offers advantages in many instances, particularly when defects are extensive or involve both hard and soft tissue. As a reflection of the invaluable utility of free tissue transfer, the number of opportunities to pursue clinical fellowship programs has grown significantly.

Originally a modality unique to plastic and reconstructive surgery (PRS), head and neck microvascular reconstruction is increasingly performed by otolaryngology (ENT) and oral and maxillofacial surgery (OMS).[2] Today, there are numerous organizations that oversee clinical fellowship training in head and neck microvascular surgery, including the Commission on Dental Accreditation, the American Head and Neck Society, the American Academy of Facial Plastic and Reconstructive Surgery, and the American Society for Reconstructive Microsurgery.[2]

Free tissue transfer in the maxillofacial region often necessitates a 2-teamed approach. The emphasis should be on the word, *team*, because both the ablative and reconstructive surgeons must work in concert toward a common goal. A critical example is the preservation of potential recipient vessels by the ablative surgeon. Although final vessel preparation is generally completed by the surgeon performing the anastomosis, an ablative surgeon's efforts to preserve and clean potential recipient vessels can make all the difference for the reconstructive surgeon. This article highlights

Disclosure: The authors have nothing to disclose.
[a] Department of Oral and Maxillofacial Surgery, The University of Texas Health Science Center at Houston, 6560 Fannin Street, Suite 1900, Houston, TX 77030, USA; [b] Head and Neck Oncologic and Microvascular Reconstructive Surgery, Providence Portland Medical Center, Portland, OR, USA
* Corresponding author.
E-mail address: jonathan.shum@uth.tmc.edu

Oral Maxillofacial Surg Clin N Am 31 (2019) 637–646
https://doi.org/10.1016/j.coms.2019.07.008

the general principles and some technical nuances involved in the preparation of neck vessels and the recipient site for successful free tissue transfer, with the goal of increasing collaboration between surgeons.

GENERAL CONSIDERATIONS

Although recipient vessels in the ipsilateral neck are most often preferred for pedicle geometry and convenience in access, the contralateral neck may be considered in cases of previous ipsilateral neck dissection. Preparation of a previously operated neck can be complicated by dense fibrotic scarring and loss of landmarks that can lead to inadvertent vessel injury. Considerations regarding the free flap pedicle orientation can also dictate the neck laterality for vascularization.

A vascular anastomosis within a previously operated neck has been associated with statistically significant increased risk of flap failure.[3] A combination of adjuvant therapy, such as radiation therapy or chemotherapy, with prior surgery can further compound the difficulties encountered and lead to increased operating time.[4] A history of radiation and/or chemotherapy has not been associated with free flap loss in the absence of previous surgery.[3–5]

Angiographic studies can guide the surgeon in salvaging vessels in a previously operated neck by confirming the location of sufficient vasculature.[5,6] In the setting of a neck that has never been operated, there is no indication for dedicated angiography to evaluate for neck vascularity.

ARTERY SELECTION

Although many factors are involved in choosing a recipient artery for each individual case, the authors generally prefer (in order) the facial artery, the superior thyroid artery (STA), and the lingual artery due to their consistent anatomic location, length and diameter of the vessel, and perfusion. These branches of the external carotid artery (ECA) are routinely encountered during ablative maxillofacial procedures, and the surgeon should be comfortable in identifying and preserving these vessels. In certain cases, the location of the flap or unsuitability of the aforementioned vessels may necessitate an alternate choice for the recipient artery. Examples include the superficial temporal artery or ECA itself via an end-to-end or end-to-side anastomosis. Some investigators have advocated for the utilization of recipient arteries outside of the external carotid system—especially in the vessel-depleted neck—which includes the transverse cervical artery, the thoracoacromial system, and the internal mammary artery.[7–9] Despite descriptions of differing qualities of the various arteries, the vessel name is less important than the quality and integrity of the individual vessel chosen, as long as general rules of pedicle handling and geometry are adhered to.

Ipsilateral upper face defects and contralateral lower face and jaw defects require a relatively long pedicle for vascularization. Often, the abundant length offered by the facial artery make it ideal for these situations or when reconstructing with a flap that has a short vascular pedicle length. Utilization of the full length of the artery may require dissection superiorly along the lateral aspect of the mandible. In reconstructions of the ipsilateral mandible, oral cavity, and oropharynx, the length of the pedicle associated with the free flap usually is adequate to access the facial artery where it protrudes from behind the posterior belly of digastric. Alternatively, the STA or lingual artery may be identified and isolated if the facial artery is not suitable. In all cases, it is desired to preserve as much recipient vessel length as possible because the flap pedicle length may be limited.

VEIN SELECTION

There are many choices for recipient veins in the neck, including the common facial vein, lingual vein, and superior thyroid vein (all tributaries of the internal jugular vein [IJV]) as well as the external jugular vein (EJV). The IJV represents the deep venous drainage pathway of the neck, whereas the EJV is a component of the superficial pathway.[10] Utilization of the anterior jugular vein is not advisable due to its trajectory near the midline of the neck, making it prone to damage in case of tracheostomy.

Commonly, the 2 veins that are identified as candidates for anastomosis include the EJV and any tributary branch to the IJV. Preference is generally given to a vein that drains into the deep (IJV) system, because the negative intrathoracic pressure produced during inspiration creates a suction effect that may assist venous outflow and prevent stasis.[11–13] **Fig. 1** demonstrates the prepared IJV with a draining tributary branch adjoining along the anterior wall of IJV. Additionally, the EJV may be more susceptible to occlusion due to improper neck position during the early postoperative course. Although several sources have reported higher rates of flap failure with EJV drainage versus the IJV, 1 study of single-vein anastomosis to the EJV demonstrated no difference compared with historical controls.[14,15] Fortunately, many of the flaps used in head and neck reconstruction carry 2 or more veins available for

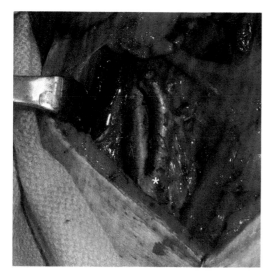

Fig. 1. A view of the carotid triangle. The IJV is prepared demonstrating the draining common facial vein tributary (*asterisk*) along the anterior wall of the IJV.

anastomosis to recipient vessels. In these cases, it is advocated to perform 2 venous anastomoses because this has been shown to decrease the risk of flap loss compared with the use of a single venous anastomosis.[16–19]

In the event there is no viable branch to the IJV, an end-to-side anastomosis to the IJV should be considered. Isolation of the IJV circumferentially for a length of 1.5 cm to 2 cm provides visualization and freedom in movement to allow for an end-to-side anastomosis.

ANATOMY AND LANDMARKS

Although there may be variations in vascular anatomy between individuals, knowledge of anatomic landmarks remains essential for identifying and preserving vessels for microvascular anastomosis.

The carotid system is the principal arterial supply encountered in resections for maxillofacial pathology. After arising from the aortic arch on the left side and the brachiocephalic artery on the right side, the common carotid artery (CCA) travels superiorly into the anterior triangle of the neck, deep/medial and anterior to the IJV. Just above the thyroid cartilage, the CCA bifurcates into the ECA and internal carotid artery (ICA).[20] The CCA and cervical portion of the ICA usually do not give off any branches, whereas the ECA gives off numerous branches to supply much of the cervical and facial tissues.

The most proximal branch of the ECA is the STA, arising just below the hyoid bone. Although it is generally depicted as a branch of the proximal ECA, the STA sometimes arises from the carotid bifurcation, the CCA, or occasionally from the ICA. The STA travels anteriorly toward the hyoid bone before descending at a steep inferior angle adjacent to the thyroid cartilage toward the midline and superior aspect of the thyroid gland, giving off several branches along the way.[21]

The lingual artery is the next most proximal anterior branch of the ECA. It may arise independently, on average 1.2 cm from the carotid bifurcation; however, in a minority of cases it arises from a shared linguofacial, thyrolingual, or thyrolingualfacial trunk. After branching from the ECA, the lingual artery briefly travels superiorly before changing course down to the greater cornu of the hyoid bone. It then resumes its superior course passing medial to the hypoglossal nerve and hyoglossus muscle. Although not encountered during routine neck dissection, the distal lingual artery may be easily revealed by dissection of the hyoglossus muscle through the Pirogoff triangle, defined within the boundaries of the posterior margin of the mylohyoid muscle, the posterior belly of the digastric muscle, and the hypoglossal nerve (**Fig. 2**).[22]

The facial artery originates from the ECA posterior to the mandibular angle, approximately 2 cm superior to the carotid bifurcation. The facial artery courses deep to the posterior belly of the digastric and along the medial aspect of the submandibular gland prior to crossing the inferior border of the mandible. It then travels along the lateral surface of the mandible superiorly before branching into the labial arteries and the angular artery. In a cadaveric study by Ozgur and colleagues,[23] the

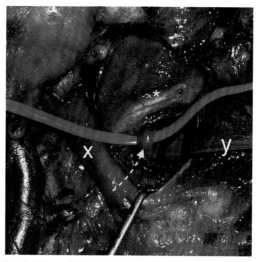

Fig. 2. Pirogoff triangle: asterisk, hypoglossal nerve; arrow, lingual artery; x, posterior belly of digastric muscle; and y, retracted mylohyoid muscle.

diameters of the superior thyroid, lingual, and facial arteries at their origins were 3.53 mm ± 1.17 mm, 3.06 mm ± 0.65 mm, and 3.35 mm ± 0.68 mm, respectively. The common branching patterns of the ECA are demonstrated in **Fig. 3**.

The venous anatomy in the neck can show considerable variation, including differing drainage pathways, as well as the number and position of venous tributaries. The EJV is the first vein encountered in dissection of the neck, due to its superficial position. The EJV originates from the union of the posterior auricular vein and the posterior division of the retromandibular vein just posterior to the angle of the mandible. It then courses inferiorly, superficial to the sternocleidomastoid muscle, prior to draining into 1 of 3 patterns: into the confluence of the subclavian vein and the IJV, into the subclavian vein itself, or rarely into the IJV.[24] There may be multiple EJVs present, or it may be absent entirely.

The IJV is the largest vein in the neck. After exiting the jugular foramen, the IJV courses down the side of the neck lateral to the ICA and CCA and deep to the sternocleidomastoid muscle before draining into the brachiocephalic vein. The IJV usually has branches only from the anterior surface, which includes the superior thyroid vein, facial vein, and lingual vein. Posterior or lateral branches, however, have been described. In rare cases the IJV may be hypoplastic or may be duplicated.[25]

VESSEL CLAMPS

To preserve as much vessel length possible, the application of a vascular occlusion clamp is preferred over a hemoclip, which necessitates truncation and further shortening if used for anastomosis. The appropriate vessel occlusion clamps are specific to the diameter of the vessel and are calibrated to be no greater than 3 times the minimum occlusive force for a vessel of that size.[26,27] Damage to the endothelium is observed when the force exceeds these defined thresholds.[26,27] Patient age, blood pressure, vessel size, wall thickness, and elasticity are several factors that influence the strength of vessels walls.[27]

Awareness of the type and specifications of the microvascular clamps is necessary to avoid inadvertent injury to the vessel and subsequent thrombosis risk. The authors prefer disposable microvascular clamps for the consistent calibrated and reliable closing pressure, antireflective surface, and availability (**Fig. 4**). Metal clamps often are reflective and carry a theoretic risk of fatigue of the metal from usage, frequent sterilization, and cleaning processes, which can alter the vascular occlusion pressure. Clamps should be placed as distal as possible along the chosen vessel. It has been reported that prolonged clamping of vessels beyond 2 hours to 3 hours may increase the rate of vessel thrombosis.[16]

VESSEL HANDLING—ARTERY

Care must be taken when isolating the vessel for anastomosis. Firstly, surgical loupe magnification and the proper instruments should be utilized when handling vessels for the purpose of dissection and isolation. Nontoothed forceps, such as DeBakey or Gerald-DeBakey, are ideal for handling the surrounding connective tissue and adventitia associated with the artery. Further isolation and dissection of the vessel are completed with an angled fine-nosed dissector, such as Dierks or McCabe. The tips of these instruments facilitate separation of the vessel from the surrounding connective tissue, and these instruments are ideal when working around small branches and tributaries. Small branches of the artery should be ligated either with surgical clips or with a bipolar

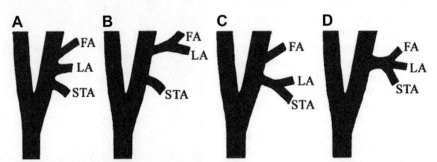

Fig. 3. The branching types of the front branches of the ECA. (*A*) STA, LA, and FA originated as separate branches (type I). (*B*) Linguofacial trunk (type II). (*C*) Thyrolingual trunk (type III). (*D*) Thyrolinguofacial trunk (type IV). FA, Facial artery; LA, Lingual artery; STA, Superior thyroid artery. (*From* Ozgur Z, Govsa F, Ozgur T. Assessment of origin characteristics of the front branches of the external carotid artery. J Craniofac Surg 2008;19(4):1159-66; with permission.)

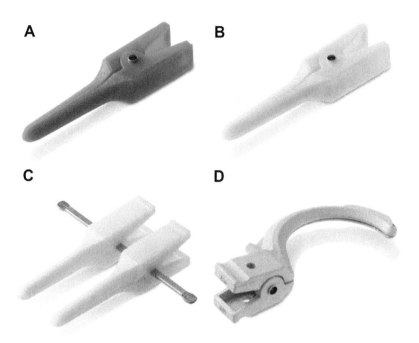

Fig. 4. (*A*) Single vein clamp. (*B*) Single artery clamp. (*C*) Double artery clamp. (*D*) End-to-side clamp. (*Courtesy of* AROSurgical, Newport Beach, CA.)

cautery prior to separation. The bipolar is used in a gentle pecking motion along the side branch away from the junction to the vessel of interest. Preferably, the side branch should be cauterized at least 2 mm away from the main vessel to prevent collateral thermal injury.[28,29]

Caution also must be taken when manipulating or retracting the vessel to facilitate dissection. Animal studies have demonstrated that excessive dissection and stretching are strong stimuli of vasospasm.[30,31] Weak stimuli for vasospasm include compressive forces from vascular clamps. The use of vessel loops for retraction or to facilitate dissection should be avoided because these may cause excessive tension that can propagate along the artery if used inappropriately.[32,33]

The length of an isolated artery necessary for anastomosis can vary and is largely based on surgeon preference. The ideal segment of an artery for anastomosis is without branches or evidence of intimal defects, such as intimal tears, calcifications, and dissection between the intima and media layers. When clinically feasible, preservation of at least of 1.0 cm of suitable artery is ideal. **Figs. 5** and **6** outline the general steps in the preparation of an artery.

When applicable to the clinical scenario, the authors prefer the facial artery to be disconnected and clipped as it curves under the inferior border of the mandible. This minimizes the risk of injury

from inadvertent traction or pressure. Within the academic setting, there are many residents, students, and teams who may be involved in a microvascular reconstruction. Inattentive and/or unfamiliar participants may traumatize a facial artery that is left in continuity over the jaw. Injury to the arterial wall, specifically the intimal lining, can lead to activation of the clotting cascade, resulting in vessel thrombosis.

VESSEL HANDLING—VEIN

Veins are inherently less robust than arteries of the same caliber. Venous walls contains relatively thin medial layers, which increases susceptibility to inadvertent damage from aggressive handling of the vessel. The use of nontoothed forceps is helpful to avoid injuries, such as perforation or aneurysm formation, due to weakening of the vein wall. Isolation of the vein is facilitated when gentle traction and counter-traction is applied to allow visualization of the interface between the wall of the vein and adjacent fascia (**Fig. 7**). Beware of small branches along the vein, because a tear would render that segment of the vein susceptible to thrombosis. Caution should be taken when dissecting along the deep surface of the vein without direct visualization, because small branches may be present in these areas. Providing gentle out-of-plane traction to the vessel can help identify

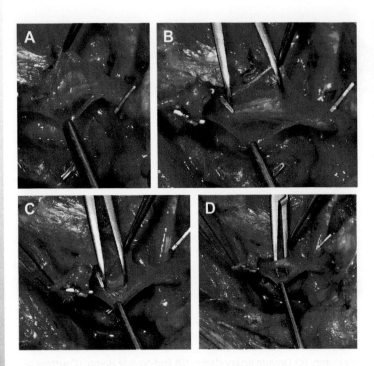

Fig. 5. (*A*) The artery is held with non-tooth forceps along the adventitia that surrounds the vessel proper. (*B*) A dissection motion parallel to the wall of the vessel is performed to remove loose connective tissue/adventitia to prepare for free tissue transfer. (*C*) The adventitia is separated along both sides of the vessel. (*D*) Circumferential dissection around the artery is completed.

deep branches that otherwise are obscured from vision. When separating the adventitial layer from the vein wall, there should be minimal effort with the dissecting forceps to open the fascial planes and expose the vein.

If ligation is required after vein preparation, a single hemoclip at the most distal extent of the vein is applied. Suture ligature is not preferred

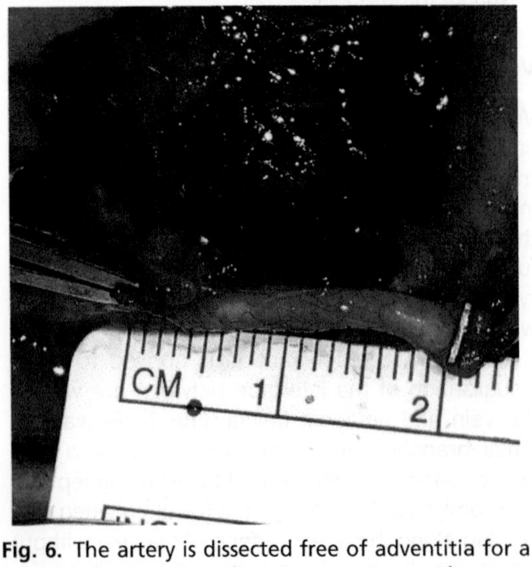

Fig. 6. The artery is dissected free of adventitia for a length of approximately 1.5 cm to 2 cm. Also note the placement of a vascular clip at the most distal site of the vessel end to preserve pedicle length.

due to the inherent constriction and traumatic shearing forces that can further foreshorten the desired vessel due to injury. Care should be taken to preserve vessel length that could be used for anastomosis.

Circumferential preparation of the IJV may be necessary if no suitable branches are identified. Dissection should proceed along the natural subfascial plane adjacent to the vein. Generally, the branches of the IJV are found exclusively along the anterior wall, because tributaries entering the IJV from the lateral, medial, or posterior are rare. Circumferential preparation allows for the application of vascular clamps, such as a small Satinsky clamp, to facilitate venotomy and anastomosis in an end-to-side fashion. Although tributary vein walls can be delicate and thin, the walls of the IJV are relatively thick and elastic and can tolerate moderate handling with a vascular forceps, such as a DeBakey. Caution should be observed with fine-tipped forceps, such as a jeweler, or with toothed forceps, because they can potentially perforate the wall of the IJV.

FINAL PREPARATION

During final preparation, the vessel is truncated just proximal to the most distal hemoclip, followed by topical heparin irrigation within the lumen and inspection for intimal defects, tears, and calcifications. Often, the isolation of approximately 15 mm to 20 mm of the vessel is sufficient to account for

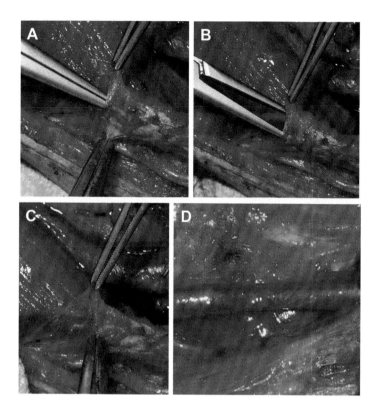

Fig. 7. (*A*) The vein is grasped with 2 nontoothed forceps to tent the overlying adventia to facilitate dissection. (*B*) A Dierk dissecting forcep is used to open the tissue plane between the vein wall and the adventitia. (*C*) The vein is exposed after careful dissection along the vein wall. (*D*) The vein is exposed along a 2-cm length, ready for anastomosis.

any additional truncation of the vessel that may be required. Again, the ideal vessel segment for anastomosis is without intimal defects, significant calcifications, or branches that are adjacent to the site of anastomosis. The presence of these features can disrupt blood flow and increase the likelihood for thrombosis.

Prior to the completion of the vascularized tissue harvest and the initiation of ischemia time, proper preparation of the recipient site vessels is verified. The surgical wound bed is irrigated with warm saline to remove debris. To ensure adequate hemostasis, a Valsalva maneuver may be performed, or the patient can be temporarily positioned in Trendelenburg.[34] The selected donor and recipient vessels should be examined to ensure a passive position, with no pressure or tension on the vessel. The intensity of blood flow is verified by briefly unclamping the vessels. A surgical sponge saturated with a vasodilator is placed over the vessels to provide both moisture and vasodilation to prevent and/or relieve vasospasm. Prolonged desiccation of the vessels should be avoided because this can lead to irreversible endothelial layer injury.[35] The authors apply an additional layer of moisture with a lap sponge saturated with warm saline to cover the entire extent of the neck wound at this time.

HEPARINIZED SALINE

Topical heparinized saline is the most commonly used irrigant during vessel preparation. Heparin binds and activates antithrombin III, leading to inhibition of several enzymatic factors in the clotting cascade.[36,37] Local irrigation with heparin has been used in various concentrations, with several studies finding 100 U/mL to be effective in reducing the risk of microvascular thrombosis while avoiding significant systemic effects.[38–40] After the application of a vascular clamp, the authors prefer a 26-gauge angiocatheter on a 10-mL syringe for gentle irrigation to remove blood and debris from within the lumen and to inspect the vessel lumen for integrity. The catheter tip need not to be placed deep into the vessel lumen. A common alternative to the angiocatheter is a vessel irrigation cannula, which utilizes a rounded blunt tip to prevent damage to the intima. Irrigation with heparinized saline is also useful in instances where there is bleeding from a potential recipient vein or artery, to assist in visualization for repair or application of a clip.

VASODILATORS

A topical vasodilator solution is often used to prevent or treat vasospasm during free flap surgery.[41] There are numerous topical agents that have been evaluated for their vasodilatory properties, including phosphodiesterase inhibitors (papaverine and pentoxifylline), local anesthetics (lidocaine), calcium channel blockers (nicardipine and verapamil), direct vasodilators (nitroglycerin), and α-antagonists (phentolamine and chlorpromazine). A survey of plastic surgeons in the United Kingdom in 2011 showed that 52% of respondents used papaverine, 47% used verapamil, and 24% used lidocaine.[41] Rationale for particular choices of topical agents was based mostly on opinions or personal experience.

The literature regarding efficacy of topical vasodilators during microsurgery is limited mostly to animal studies and in vitro experiments on human vessels.[42] These studies give insight into notable differences in the physiologic effects of the various agents. For example, papaverine has shown efficacy as a vasodilator in many studies; however, it has also been shown to cause endothelial damage in in vitro studies.[43] Although lidocaine has shown significant vasodilation at high concentrations (12%–20%), in lower concentrations (1%–2%) lidocaine actually produces vasoconstriction in most animal models.[44,45] Several other agents, such as nicardipine, magnesium sulfate, and phentolamine, have shown promising activity in animal studies but have limited evidence for use in microvascular surgery.[42]

Although consensus on the ideal topical agent has yet to be reached, the choice of which agent to use may be of minimal consequence. Studies of flap outcomes during a papaverine shortage showed no increase in flap failure with use of lidocaine, nicardipine, or nitroglycerin when compared with papaverine historical controls.[46,47]

APPLICATIONS IN ORAL AND MAXILLOFACIAL SURGERY

As the specialty of OMS continues to evolve, the utilization of microvascular techniques in OMS programs will continue to become more common. Whether related to the influx of microvascular-trained OMS in academic centers or to collaborative efforts with plastic and reconstructive surgery or otolaryngology, the likelihood of participating in a case utilizing microvascular reconstruction is increasingly likely. Therefore, ensuring familiarity with basic vessel handling techniques is to the benefit of patients and one's microvascular colleagues. By learning the key principles of vessel preservation, all involved surgeons can avoid potential pitfalls and move toward the common goal of successful reconstruction.

Prior to microvascular reconstructive cases, a preoperative discussion with the reconstructive

surgeon should occur. The management of the recipient vessels is technique sensitive, and preference on how to isolate and prepare the vessels may vary. All efforts should be made to handle the vasculature with care and to avoid inadvertent traction or direct manipulation of the vessel walls. Due to a pathology or a traumatic defect, the desired blood vessel may be truncated, and attempts to preserve every millimeter of the vessel should be made. An understanding of the techniques and anatomic landmarks outlined in this article will provide a foundation for safe vessel handling and preparation of vessels for microvascular anastomosis.

REFERENCES

1. Shah J. A century of progress in head and neck cancer. J Head Neck Physicians Surg 2016;4(2):50–8.
2. Markiewicz MR, Miloro M. The evolution of microvascular and microneurosurgical maxillofacial reconstruction. J Oral Maxillofac Surg 2018;76(4):687–99.
3. Mucke T, Rau A, Weitz J, et al. Influence of irradiation and oncologic surgery on head and neck microsurgical reconstructions. Oral Oncol 2012;48(4):367–71.
4. Rostetter C, Kuster IM, Schenkel JS, et al. The effects of preoperative radiotherapy on head and neck free flap anastomosis success. J Oral Maxillofac Surg 2016;74(12):2521–5.
5. Hanasono MM, Barnea Y, Skoracki RJ. Microvascular surgery in the previously operated and irradiated neck. Microsurgery 2009;29(1):1–7.
6. Jones NF, Jarrahy R, Song JI, et al. Postoperative medical complications–not microsurgical complications–negatively influence the morbidity, mortality, and true costs after microsurgical reconstruction for head and neck cancer. Plast Reconstr Surg 2007;119(7):2053–60.
7. Harris JR, Lueg E, Genden E, et al. The thoracoacromial/cephalic vascular system for microvascular anastomoses in the vessel-depleted neck. Arch Otolaryngol Head Neck Surg 2002;128(3):319–23.
8. Yu P. The transverse cervical vessels as recipient vessels for previously treated head and neck cancer patients. Plast Reconstr Surg 2005;115(5):1253–8.
9. Buck PM, Wax MK, Petrisor DI. Internal mammary vessels: alternate recipient vessels in microvascular head and neck reconstruction. J Oral Maxillofac Surg 2016;74(9):1896.e1-6.
10. Asouhidou I, Natsis K, Asteri T, et al. Anatomical variation of left internal jugular vein: clinical significance for an anaesthesiologist. Eur J Anaesthesiol 2008;25(4):314–8.
11. Wax MK, Quraishi H, Rodman S, et al. Internal jugular vein patency in patients undergoing

microvascular reconstruction. Laryngoscope 1997;
107(9):1245–8.

12. Ueda K, Harii K, Nakatsuka T, et al. Comparison of
    end-to-end and end-to-side venous anastomosis in
    free-tissue transfer following resection of head and
    neck tumors. Microsurgery 1996;17(3):146–9.

13. Chia HL, Wong CH, Tan BK, et al. An algorithm for
    recipient vessel selection in microsurgical head
    and neck reconstruction. J Reconstr Microsurg
    2011;27(1):47–56.

14. Hong P, Taylor SM, Trites JR, et al. Use of the
    external jugular vein as the sole recipient vein
    in head and neck free flap reconstruction.
    J Otolaryngol 2006;35(6):361–5.

15. Chalian AA, Anderson TD, Weinstein GS, et al. Inter-
    nal jugular vein versus external jugular vein anasta-
    mosis: implications for successful free tissue
    transfer. Head Neck 2001;23(6):475–8.

16. Braun SA, Mine R, Syed SA, et al. The optimal
    sequence of microvascular repair during prolonged
    clamping in free flap transfer. Plast Reconstr Surg
    2003;111(1):233–41.

17. Zhang T, Lubek J, Salama A, et al. Venous anasto-
    moses using microvascular coupler in free flap
    head and neck reconstruction. J Oral Maxillofac
    Surg 2012;70(4):992–6.

18. Riot S, Herlin C, Mojallal A, et al. A systematic review
    and meta-analysis of double venous anastomosis
    in free flaps. Plast Reconstr Surg 2015;136(6):
    1299–311.

19. Chaput B, Vergez S, Somda S, et al. comparison of
    single and double venous anastomoses in head and
    neck oncologic reconstruction using free flaps: a
    meta-analysis. Plast Reconstr Surg 2016;137(5):
    1583–94.

20. Riberio RA, Ribeiro JAS, Rodrigues Filho OA, et al.
    Common Carotid Artery Bifurcation Levels Related
    to Clinical Relevant Anatomical Landmarks. Int J
    Morphol 2006;24(3):413–6.

21. Won SY. Anatomical considerations of the superior
    thyroid artery: its origins, variations, and position
    relative to the hyoid bone and thyroid cartilage.
    Anat Cell Biol 2016;49(2):138–42.

22. van Es RJ, Thuau H. Pirogoff's Triangle revisited: an
    alternative site for microvascular anastomosis to the
    lingual artery. A technical note. Int J Oral Maxillofac
    Surg 2000;29(3):207–9.

23. Ozgur Z, Govsa F, Ozgur T. Assessment of origin
    characteristics of the front branches of the external
    carotid artery. J Craniofac Surg 2008;19(4):1159–66.

24. Kopuz C, Akan H. The importance of the angulation
    and termination of external jugular vein in central
    venous catheterization in newborn. Okajimas Folia
    Anat Jpn 1996;73(2–3):155–9.

25. Deepak CA, Sarvadnya JJ, Sabitha KS. Variant anat-
    omy of internal jugular vein branching. Ann Maxillo-
    fac Surg 2015;5(2):284–6.

26. Trobec R, Gersak B. Direct measurement of clamp-
    ing forces in cardiovascular surgery. Med Biol Eng
    Comput 1997;35(1):17–20.

27. Sauer CM, Tomlin DH, Mozaffari Naeini H, et al.
    Real-time measurement of blood vessel occlusion
    during microsurgery. Comput Aided Surg 2002;
    7(6):364–70.

28. Hood JM, Lubahn JD. Bipolar coagulation at
    different energy levels: effect on patency. Microsur-
    gery 1994;15(8):594–7.

29. Caffee HH, Ward D. Bipolar coagulation in microvas-
    cular surgery. Plast Reconstr Surg 1986;78(3):
    374–7.

30. Hyza P, Streit L, Schwarz D, et al. Vasospasm of the
    flap pedicle - the new experimental model on rat.
    Acta Chir Plast 2014;56(1–2):3–11.

31. Hyza P, Vesely J, Schwarz D, et al. The effect of
    blood around a flap pedicle on flap perfusion in an
    experimental rodent model. Acta Chir Plast 2009;
    51(1):21–5.

32. Bunt TJ, Manship L, Moore W. Iatrogenic vascular
    injury during peripheral revascularization. J Vasc
    Surg 1985;2(3):491–8.

33. Slayback JB, Bowen WW, Hinshaw DB. Intimal
    injury from arterial clamps. Am J Surg 1976;
    132(2):183–8.

34. Moumoulidis I, Martinez Del Pero M, Brennan L,
    et al. Haemostasis in head and neck surgical pro-
    cedures: Valsalva manoeuvre versus Trendelenburg
    tilt. Ann R Coll Surg Engl 2010;92(4):292–4.

35. Acland RD. Microvascular anastomosis: a device for
    holding stay sutures and a new vascular clamp. Sur-
    gery 1974;75(2):185–7.

36. Rhee RY, Donayre CE, Ouriel K, et al. Low dose hep-
    arin therapy: in vitro verification of antithrombotic ef-
    fect. J Vasc Surg 1991;14(5):628–34.

37. Johnson PC, Barker JH. Thrombosis and antithrom-
    botic therapy in microvascular surgery. Clin Plast
    Surg 1992;19(4):799–807.

38. Andresen DM, Barker JH, Hjortdal VE. Local heparin
    is superior to systemic heparin in preventing arterial
    thrombosis. Microsurgery 2002;22(6):265–72.

39. Cox GW, Runnels S, Hsu HS, et al. A comparison of
    heparinised saline irrigation solutions in a model of
    microvascular thrombosis. Br J Plast Surg 1992;
    45(5):345–8.

40. Couteau C, Rem K, Guillier D, et al. Improving free-
    flap survival using intra-operative heparin: Ritualistic
    practice or evidence-base medicine? A systematic
    review. Ann Chir Plast Esthet 2018;63(3):e1–5.

41. Yu JT, Patel AJ, Malata CM. The use of topical vaso-
    dilators in microvascular surgery. J Plast Reconstr
    Aesthet Surg 2011;64(2):226–8.

42. Vargas CR, Iorio ML, Lee BT. A systematic review of
    topical vasodilators for the treatment of intraopera-
    tive vasospasm in reconstructive microsurgery. Plast
    Reconstr Surg 2015;136(2):411–22.

43. Gao YJ, Yang H, Teoh K, et al. Detrimental effects of papaverine on the human internal thoracic artery. J Thorac Cardiovasc Surg 2003;126(1):179–85.

44. Evans GR, Gherardini G, Gurlek A, et al. Drug-induced vasodilation in an in vitro and in vivo study: the effects of nicardipine, papaverine, and lidocaine on the rabbit carotid artery. Plast Reconstr Surg 1997;100(6):1475–81.

45. Gherardini G, Gurlek A, Cromeens D, et al. Drug-induced vasodilation: in vitro and in vivo study on the effects of lidocaine and papaverine on rabbit carotid artery. Microsurgery 1998;18(2):90–6.

46. Ricci JA, Koolen PG, Shah J, et al. Comparing the outcomes of different agents to treat vasospasm at microsurgical anastomosis during the papaverine shortage. Plast Reconstr Surg 2016;138(3):401e–8e.

47. Ricci JA, Singhal D, Fukudome EY, et al. Topical nitroglycerin for the treatment of intraoperative microsurgical vasospasm. Microsurgery 2018; 38(5):524–9.

UNITED STATES POSTAL SERVICE® Statement of Ownership, Management, and Circulation (All Periodicals Publications Except Requester Publications)

1. Publication Title	2. Publication Number	3. Filing Date
ORAL & MAXILLOFACIAL SURGERY CLINICS OF NORTH AMERICA	006 – 362	9/18/2019

4. Issue Frequency	5. Number of Issues Published Annually	6. Annual Subscription Price
FEB, MAY, AUG, NOV	4	$401.00

7. Complete Mailing Address of Known Office of Publication (Not printer) (Street, city, county, state, and ZIP+4®)

ELSEVIER INC.
230 Park Avenue, Suite 800
New York, NY 10169

Contact Person
STEPHEN R. BUSHING

Telephone (Include area code)
215-239-3688

8. Complete Mailing Address of Headquarters or General Business Office of Publisher (Not printer)

ELSEVIER INC.
230 Park Avenue, Suite 800
New York, NY 10169

9. Full Names and Complete Mailing Addresses of Publisher, Editor, and Managing Editor (Do not leave blank)

Publisher (Name and complete mailing address)

TAYLOR BALL, ELSEVIER INC.
1600 JOHN F KENNEDY BLVD. SUITE 1800
PHILADELPHIA, PA 19103-2899

Editor (Name and complete mailing address)

JOHN VASSALLO, ELSEVIER INC.
1600 JOHN F KENNEDY BLVD. SUITE 1800
PHILADELPHIA, PA 19103-2899

Managing Editor (Name and complete mailing address)

PATRICK MANLEY, ELSEVIER INC.
1600 JOHN F KENNEDY BLVD. SUITE 1800
PHILADELPHIA, PA 19103-2899

10. Owner (Do not leave blank. If the publication is owned by a corporation, give the name and address of the corporation immediately followed by the names and addresses of all stockholders owning or holding 1 percent or more of the total amount of stock. If not owned by a corporation, give the names and addresses of the individual owners. If owned by a partnership or other unincorporated firm, give its name and address as well as those of each individual owner. If the publication is published by a nonprofit organization, give its name and address.)

Full Name	Complete Mailing Address
WHOLLY OWNED SUBSIDIARY OF REED/ELSEVIER, US HOLDINGS	1600 JOHN F KENNEDY BLVD. SUITE 1800 PHILADELPHIA, PA 19103-2899

11. Known Bondholders, Mortgagees, and Other Security Holders Owning or Holding 1 Percent or More of Total Amount of Bonds, Mortgages, or Other Securities. If none, check box ▶ ☐ None

Full Name	Complete Mailing Address
N/A	

12. Tax Status (For completion by nonprofit organizations authorized to mail at nonprofit rates) (Check one)
The purpose, function, and nonprofit status of this organization and the exempt status for federal income tax purposes:
☒ Has Not Changed During Preceding 12 Months
☐ Has Changed During Preceding 12 Months (Publisher must submit explanation of change with this statement)

PS Form 3526, July 2014 (Page 1 of 4 (see instructions page 4)) PSN: 7530-01-000-9931

---

13. Publication Title		14. Issue Date for Circulation Data Below
ORAL & MAXILLOFACIAL SURGERY CLINICS OF NORTH AMERICA		AUGUST 2019

15. Extent and Nature of Circulation			Average No. Copies Each Issue During Preceding 12 Months	No. Copies of Single Issue Published Nearest to Filing Date
a. Total Number of Copies (Net press run)			568	667
b. Paid Circulation (By Mail and Outside the Mail)	(1)	Mailed Outside-County Paid Subscriptions Stated on PS Form 3541 (Include paid distribution above nominal rate, advertiser's proof copies, and exchange copies)	430	446
	(2)	Mailed In-County Paid Subscriptions Stated on PS Form 3541 (Include paid distribution above nominal rate, advertiser's proof copies, and exchange copies)	0	0
	(3)	Paid Distribution Outside the Mails Including Sales Through Dealers and Carriers, Street Vendors, Counter Sales, and Other Paid Distribution Outside USPS®	72	73
	(4)	Paid Distribution by Other Classes of Mail Through the USPS (e.g. First-Class Mail®)	0	0
c. Total Paid Distribution (Sum of 15b (1), (2), (3), and (4))		▶	502	519
d. Free or Nominal Rate Distribution (By Mail and Outside the Mail)	(1)	Free or Nominal Rate Outside-County Copies included on PS Form 3541	52	130
	(2)	Free or Nominal Rate In-County Copies Included on PS Form 3541	0	0
	(3)	Free or Nominal Rate Copies Mailed at Other Classes Through the USPS (e.g. First-Class Mail)	0	0
	(4)	Free or Nominal Rate Distribution Outside the Mail (Carriers or other means)	0	0
e. Total Free or Nominal Rate Distribution (Sum of 15d (1), (2), (3) and (4))		▶	52	130
f. Total Distribution (Sum of 15c and 15e)		▶	554	649
g. Copies not Distributed (See Instructions to Publishers #4 (page #3))		▶	14	18
h. Total (Sum of 15f and g)		▶	568	667
i. Percent Paid (15c divided by 15f times 100)		▶	77.62%	79.97%

* If you are claiming electronic copies, go to line 16 on page 3. If you are not claiming electronic copies, skip to line 17 on page 3.

16. Electronic Copy Circulation		Average No. Copies Each Issue During Preceding 12 Months	No. Copies of Single Issue Published Nearest to Filing Date
a. Paid Electronic Copies	▶		
b. Total Paid Print Copies (Line 15c) + Paid Electronic Copies (Line 16a)	▶		
c. Total Print Distribution (Line 15f) + Paid Electronic Copies (Line 16a)	▶		
d. Percent Paid (Both Print & Electronic Copies) (16b divided by 16c × 100)	▶		

☒ I certify that 50% of all my distributed copies (electronic and print) are paid above a nominal price.

17. Publication of Statement of Ownership
☒ If the publication is a general publication, publication of this statement is required. Will be printed in the NOVEMBER 2019 issue of this publication. ☐ Publication not required.

18. Signature and Title of Editor, Publisher, Business Manager, or Owner

STEPHEN R. BUSHING - INVENTORY DISTRIBUTION CONTROL MANAGER

Stephen R. Bushing   Date 9/18/2019

I certify that all information furnished on this form is true and complete. I understand that anyone who furnishes false or misleading information on this form or who omits material or information requested on the form may be subject to criminal sanctions (including fines and imprisonment) and/or civil sanctions (including civil penalties).

PS Form 3526, July 2014 (Page 3 of 4)

Printed and bound by CPI Group (UK) Ltd, Croydon, CR0 4YY

08/05/2025

01864747-0010